The King of Herbs

This amazing tonic herb has been regarded as a "cure-all" in Asia for centuries, promising those benefits we all strive for: increased mental and physical vitality and emotional balance. More than 3,000 scientific studies attest to these health-giving properties:

- Counters stress
- Enhances immunity
- Tones the heart and lungs
- Regulates blood pressure and blood sugar
- Protects the liver
- Serves as a powerful antioxidant

About the Author

Kathi Keville is a prominent American herbalist who has been working with herbs since 1969. Her books include *Herbs: An Illustrated Encyclopedia of Herbs, Herbs: American Country Living, Aromatherapy: The Complete Guide to the Healing Art, Herbs for Health and Healing* and *Pocket Aromatherapy Guide.* She has also contributed to eight other herb books, written over 100 herb articles for national magazines, and was Associate Editor for *Well-Being* Magazine. She has lectured throughout the United States, and has been on the staff of 10 teaching institutes. Kathi is director of the American Herb Association and editor of the *AHA Quarterly*, a founding member of the American Herbalist Guild, an honorary member of the National Association of Holistic Aromatherapy and the American Aromatherapy Association. Kathi has operated an herb farm which grew and sold 400 different species of herbs for 14 years and now owns an herbal mail-order business.

A KEATS GOOD HERB GUIDE

MEDICINE
21 CENTURY

GINSENG

Kathi Keville

Keats Publishing, Inc.   New Canaan, Connecticut

GINSENG

Copyright © 1996 by Kathi Keville

All Rights Reserved

No part of this book may be reproduced in any form without the written consent of the publisher.

Library of Congress Cataloging-in-Publication Data

Keville, Kathy.
    Ginseng / by Kathi Keville.
      p.   cm.
    Includes bibliographical references and index.
    ISBN 0-87983-731-4
    1. Ginseng—Therapeutic use.   I. Title.
  RM666.G49K48 1996
  615'.323687—dc20   96-35929
                                     CIP

Printed in the United States of America

Keats Good Health Guides are published by
Keats Publishing, Inc.
27 Pine Street (Box 876)
New Canaan, Connecticut 06840-0876

98 97 96   6 5 4 3 2 1

Contents

❊❧ INTRODUCTION ❧❊

Ginseng is often called "the King of Herbs," and has been highly regarded in Asia for centuries. Its fame has spread throughout the world. The reason is simple: ginseng's age-old reputation for improving physical energy, making the mind sharper and increasing life span. Ginseng potentially offers what we all strive for—vitality, unlimited energy, intelligence and longevity. Yet, unlike popular stimulants, such as coffee or drugs containing amphetamines, it does not wreak havoc with the adrenal glands and the rest of the body. Instead, it counters stress, enhances immunity, improves the actions of the heart and lungs, regulates blood pressure and blood sugar, protects the liver, helps prevent hardening of the arteries and is an antioxidant. Summed up, it is a tonic that improves general health.

If ever an herb was considered a cure-all or panacea, ginseng is the most likely candidate. Even its botanical name, *Panax,* means "all-cure" in Greek, reflecting the ancient belief that it is a panacea. How can one herb do so much? Herbalists throughout the ages and, more lately, scientists have asked this very question. Although ginseng is well studied, with approximately 3,000 scientific studies to its credit, it is also very complex. We still do not understand exactly how it works. What we do know is that ginseng reduces stress and brings the body into balance. We also know that it is safe to take and that it provides millions of people with benefits.

Ginseng grows wild in two parts of the world: Asia and North America. In both places, the mystique of it as a panacea is enhanced by its peculiar shape. After several years' growth, the pale root that emerges when dug from the ground typically has two long leg-like roots dangling from a main torso and side roots that resemble arms with thin, long fingers. In short, the shape of the root is like a person. This fact did not escape the imagination of the ancients and still prompts an uncanny fascination with ginseng. Even the name ginseng means "essence of the earth in the form of a man." (In Chinese, *gin* is "man" and *seng* is a fleshy root used as a tonic.) Native American Cherokee also called the root "little men," or *yunwiya usdi,* and both cultures considered it sacred. Many an ancient Chinese went on a spiritual quest to find *Tu Ching,* the Spirit of the Ground, and recited an ancient chant before digging the roots.

O great spirit! Do not go away
I have come with a clean heart
My soul is unstained
It is purged of sin and wicked design
Remain here, O greatest of spirits
    —Ancient Chinese prayer to the jen-shen root

🌿 HISTORY 🌿

The history of ginseng is a rich one. A Chinese myth thought to be 2500 years old tells of digging the roots. The first mention of ginseng's miraculous powers is in China's first herb book, the *Pen Tsao-Ching,* attributed to Shen-Nung. Written in the first century A.D., the original text is much older. It recommends ginseng not only for a long life, but also for a wise one. It suggests that it be taken continuously for optimum results. Harvard botanist Shiu Ying Hu translates the description of ginseng in this ancient text as, "It is used for repairing the five viscera, quieting the spirit, curbing the emotion, stopping agitation, removing noxious influence, brightening the eyes, enlightening the mind and increasing wisdom."

Ginseng's modern history began with Father Jartoux, a Jesuit missionary stationed in China. He was mapping an area near the Chinese-Korean border for the Chinese Emperor Kanghi when he first came across ginseng and became fascinated with it. He ran into some of the emperor's ginseng collectors who brought him a basket containing four ginseng roots. Jartoux tried the curious, man-shaped roots and their effect impressed him; his pulse increased and he noticed that he had more energy. In 1714, his writings and a detailed drawing were published as *The Description of the Tartarian Plant, Gin-seng.* In it, he described how ginseng could help even healthy people stay vigorous and strong. The missionary also suggested that it would be an excellent addition to the European pharmacy and wrote, "Nobody can imagine that the Chinese and Tartars would set so high a value on this root, if it did not constantly produce a good effect." After describing how the plant loves to grow in mountain forests, he prophetically added, "All of which makes me believe that if it is to be found in any other country in the world, it may be particularly in Canada, where the forest and mountains . . . very much resemble these here.''

A year later, another Jesuit missionary, Father Joseph Francis Lafitau, read these words, and took notice. Lafitau lived north of Montreal, Canada, where he was working with the Mohawk Indians. When he showed them the drawing of ginseng, they recognized the plant and promised to find some. Three months later, he excitedly sent samples of the roots to Father Jartoux, who presented them to Chinese ginseng traders. The merchants confirmed that it was ginseng—and worth its weight in gold.

Only four years after Jartoux's publication, the first American ginseng—in fact the first of any American herb—was exported to China. The Chinese welcomed American ginseng with open arms. After centuries of collecting their own wild ginseng, it was becoming scarce. Besides, ginseng from America was a novelty. Oriental practitioners determined that the root was similar to their ginseng, but it had different ''energetic'' properties according to their system of medicine.

Early North American pioneers could not have been happier to learn that there was a valuable plant that grew as a weed in the wilderness they loved. Fur traders, already trading with Native Americans in the areas where ginseng grew wild, quickly expanded their business to include ginseng, known as 'shang. Daniel Boone was one of America's more famous 'shang traders and made most of his money from ginseng.

While American ginseng was a big hit in China, it never became important to North American physicians, who were unfamiliar with its properties. Physicians of that era had little time for a general tonic reputed to make people healthier. Instead, they used laxative purges, diuretics and plants and minerals that made their patients vomit and produced quick and impressive results. While Native Americans did regard ginseng as medicine, it was apparently never with the passion of the Orientals. However, it is debatable how widespread the Indians' use of ginseng really was until 'shang traders made it famous by selling it to China.

Ginseng did find its way into the *U.S. Pharmacopoeia*, the official book of medicine, from 1842 until 1882. It described ginseng as a stimulant and a stomachic, which is a substance that aids digestion. During this time, pharmaceutical studies began on ginseng. The first report on its chemistry was published in 1854 in the *Annals of Chemical Pharmacy*. A few studies followed, but U.S. interest in the root remained low.

Not so in Russia and Japan, the two countries that conducted most of the early ginseng research. In 1859, a Russian scientific expedition departed St. Petersburg and traveled into the Manchurian territory and the Korean frontier in search of ginseng. They knew China was importing tons of U.S. ginseng and they wanted to establish their own large plantations in Russia to sell roots to China. Research stepped up when Japan annexed Korea and later occupied ginseng-rich Manchuria and continued until the Sino-Japanese War in 1936 and World War II brought it to a halt.

Ginseng investigation again picked up in 1949 with Professor Israel I. Brekhman from the recently established Institute of Biologically Active Substances of the USSR's Academy of Sciences in Vladivostok, Siberia. The institute's mission was to explore medicinally useful herbs from China and Siberia. Its particular interest was ginseng. Brekhman observed that "Ginseng has been used as a remedy for 5,000 years. During those 50 centuries, numerous generations, social systems, medical doctrines, and medicines have sunk into oblivion, yet, ginseng still exists. It exists despite the fact that science not only ignored, but rejected it. . . ." During the next 16 years, the center made up for those years of neglect. It coordinated research from major scientific institutions throughout the USSR. It also sponsored 23 international sessions and published seven volumes of reports. All of this helped make ginseng the most extensively studied of any herb.

✺ MEET THE GINSENGS ✺

Botanically speaking, ginseng is in the *Panax* genus. The family is *Araliaceae,* which is also known as the ginseng family. There are several different species, all bearing the common name ginseng.

GINSENG (*Panax ginseng*). The best known of the clan is simply called ginseng, or sometimes Oriental, Chinese or most often, Korean ginseng to differentiate it from American ginseng. Most of the studies have been done with this species. Researchers say that the studies also apply to American ginseng, since the two are so similar in appearance and chemistry that even they have difficulty telling them apart. Chinese see it differently. They say the two species have different energetic properties and classify them as two separate types.

AMERICAN GINSENG (*Panax quinquefolius*). American ginseng grows wild from Quebec and Manitoba, Canada, south to Alabama, Oklahoma and even Florida, what little is left in the wild. Indians in these areas used it medicinally to treat indigestion, sore eyes and earache, menstrual cramps, fever and bronchitis. Iroquois warriors carried the root as a talisman and used it to offset ''old year's fire.'' Most American ginseng is cultivated in Wisconsin and Canada and shipped to the Orient. The U.S. exports over two million pounds of it a year. That totaled almost 100 million dollars in 1993. About one-fifth of this comes from the world's largest ginseng grower, a Canadian company, Chai-Na-Ta Corporation in British Columbia.

DWARF GINSENG (*Panax trifolius*). Dwarf ginseng is an American ginseng that is not very common. It grows mostly in the southern Appalachians, although its range extends from Nova Scotia to Georgia. American Indians used the root to treat headaches and nervous conditions and the whole plant for colic, cough, debility, indigestion, gout, hepatitis, hives, rheumatism and skin problems. Its globe-like, edible root gives it another name, groundnut.

SANCHI GINSENG (*Panax notoginseng*, also called *Panax pseudoginseng* variety *notoginseng*). Another

Asian ginseng is *sanch'i* or *tiench'i* ginseng (sometimes spelled *sanqi* and *tienqi*). The name means "seven" and comes from the fact that this ginseng plant has seven leaflets instead of *Panax ginseng's* five. It still grows wild and is cultivated in China's Yunnan province. Its other common names are pseudo-ginseng or noto-ginseng, since the root and the flower blossoms are sometimes used in place of *Panax ginseng* as a tonic, but it is not considered an adaptogen. Instead, Chinese hospitals use it in emergencies to stop bleeding, reduce pain, decrease swelling and move blood away from the injury—uses recorded in the ancient *Pen Tsao Kang-mu*. It is also a standard treatment for excessive blood loss or when there is blood in the urine or lungs. There is more on sanchi properties in the section on heart and circulation (see page 34).

HIMALAYAN GINSENG (*Panax pseudoginseng* subsp. *himalaicus*). This subspecies from Tibet and western Bhutan is rarely available in North America. The ginsenoside content—the amount of active medicine it contains—falls in between that of Korean and Japanese ginseng. Some botanists prefer classifying the subspecies as *japonica*.

JAPANESE GINSENG (*Panax japonicus*). The Japanese call their native ginseng *chikusetsu* and have long substituted it for *Panax ginseng* in their formulas. Japanese medical scholar Yoshimasu Todo suggested in his eighteenth century book *Yakucho* that both ginsengs be used interchangeably. Above ground, the two plants are so similar that most people cannot tell the difference. However, Japanese ginseng has a rhizome with a mass of roots extending from it, instead of being shaped like a man. In the 1920s, Japanese researchers discovered that their ginseng has similar components to *Panax ginseng,* but in different proportions that varied according to where the root grew. Chinese herbalists call this ginseng *zhu-ji-shen* and consider it less powerful than *Panax ginseng,* but therefore valuable for people who are too weak to take ginseng. They mainly use it to treat heart palpitations, fluid around the heart, lung congestion, and digestive problems, such as nausea and poor appetite. It also lowers fevers. Two more varieties named *major* and *bipinnatifidus* are an official medicine known as *zhu-zi-shen* in the Chinese pharmacopoeia, used to treat coughs and asthma.

SIBERIAN GINSENG (*Eleutherococcus senticosus*). Like ginseng, Siberian ginseng belongs to the *Araliaceae* family, but is not a true ginseng of the *Panax* genus. It is a much larger bush. As you might have guessed, it is native to Siberia. *Senticosus* describes the very prickly stems. Its properties and uses are similar to ginseng, but using the same common name for both herbs has created much confusion. For clarification, herbalists often refer to Siberian ginseng by its botanical name, *Eleutherococcus,* or simply the abbreviated "eleuthero." In each chapter of this book, Siberian ginseng appears in a separate section after true ginseng. This makes it easy for you to compare the similarities and differences and decide which one to take.

Siberian ginseng has long been used as a medicine

in China, but not with the popularity of *Panax ginseng*. In his ancient *Pen Tsao-Ching,* Shen Nung said it increases energy and treats rheumatism. The Chinese also prescribe it for weak or debilitated conditions and to improve general health. They traditionally used the root bark; nevertheless, Soviet research now shows that the whole root is more effective. Although the plant grows far into Siberia, there is no record of its use in Russia.

Modern research on Siberian ginseng began when ginseng researcher Professor Israel I. Brekhman searched the *Araliaceae* family for a ginseng substitute that grew more abundantly in Russia. The story is that one day a young Russian doctor, Nickolay Suprunov, observed a deer eating the bush in the wild and became curious about its properties. When tested, it proved to be the plant for which Brekhman was searching.

Brekhman published the first scientific findings on Siberian ginseng in 1958 and The Pharmacological Committee of the USSR (the Soviet equivalent of the FDA in the U.S.) granted permission to begin clinic tests the next year. In 1961, Brekhman's Institute of Biologically Active Substances prepared an 86-page report on Siberian ginseng and a series of symposiums. Six years later, over 80 scientific articles had been published in Russia and the herb had been tested in over 100 Soviet hospitals and clinics. Brekhman felt that Siberian ginseng has some advantages over ginseng; it lasts longer and is more calming, so hyperactive individuals who normally could not take ginseng can use it.

Siberian ginseng quickly captured the attention of the general public as a less expensive alternative to ginseng. During the 1960s, Russians went though more than 100 tons of Siberian ginseng roots a year. It went into food and several perfumes and even flavored a cola-like drink named Bordrust, meaning "vigor." The soft drink was so popular that the manufacturer could not keep up with the demand. Siberian ginseng is also added to a vodka sold as *zolotoy rog.* Although the color and taste are changed, people drink it because it reduces the intensity of a hangover. The leaves and branches of Siberian ginseng even went into animal food. The Chinese also became more interested in the plant. They added it to their *Pharmacopoeia* in 1977 and held a special symposium on it in Harbin, China the next year.

Siberian ginseng eventually made its way into the Soviet space program and through this channel found its way to the U.S. While he was lecturing at the School of Aerospace Medicine at Brooks Air Force Base in 1962, Bruce Halstead, M.D. was shown an English translation of a paper entitled, "A Rival of Ginseng," by Boris Sadekov. Halstead contacted Brekhman to learn more about the mysterious nontoxic stimulant used by cosmonauts and was invited to come to Russia to see for himself. His trip there resulted in a book, *Siberian Ginseng: An Introduction to the Concept of Adaptogenic Medicine,* about Brekhman's work.

❧ GINSENG'S CHEMISTRY ❧

The research on ginseng is extensive, yet it is hindered by ginseng itself. An herb that brings the body into balance and does so by regulating several systems in the body cannot be computed by the precise scientific mind. To complicate things more, ginseng can raise a factor, such as blood pressure or sugar, in one person, then turn around and lower it in another. Put ginseng in the body and it equals balance, but try to run these results through a computer and they do not make sense.

There are other problems facing ginseng research. For one thing, the East and West do not approach science with the same criteria. Most of the studies on ginseng and Siberian ginseng are from Russia and China and do not always meet the strict guidelines laid down by Western researchers. As a result, some Western researchers claim that there is little scientific evidence to support ginseng's use. Also, the bulk of research is on animals. Since animals' systems differ from those of people, results from these studies must be considered preliminary. Also, most of these studies used large amounts of ginseng that were given by injection. These are two factors that produce different results from normal use.

Most studies quoted in this book are the double-blind, placebo-controlled, clinical studies that are esteemed by Western scientists. This means that some participants were given ginseng while others got a dummy version without ginseng, but no one knows who had which one, often even the researchers themselves. The results are then compared to see who got the best score on whatever was tested.

Researchers are always interested in identifying and isolating a medicinal plant's active ingredient. Although ginseng does contain other compounds, science considers substances called ginsenosides responsible for most of its medicinal properties. The term "ginsenoside" was coined by Dr. Shoji Shibata at the University of Tokyo while he was studying their individual actions in 1961, but some old studies refer to them as panaxosides. They are a type of saponin, which is a group of complex carbohydrates found throughout the plant kingdom. However, ginsenosides occur only in the true *Panax* ginsengs. At last count, at least 11 important ginsenosides have been discovered in ginseng, along with about 19 others thought to be less significant.[1]

The ginsenosides cause different reactions. Some enhance muscle tone, others regulate blood sugar, and yet others stimulate the central nervous system. American ginseng has the same number of ginsenosides as Oriental ginseng, but they appear in larger quantities and in slightly different proportions, making them less stimulating. Assays also find more ginsenosides in wild American ginseng than in the cultivated roots. Each ginsenoside has its own name, with the two most important ones being called Rg1 and Rb1. Chances are, like the constituents of most herbs, they work better together than when used separately. If you want to learn more about ginseng's chemistry, consult the technical books listed in the bibliography.

The amount and proportion of ginsenosides changes depending on the species of ginseng. Even the age of the plant when harvested and where it grew alters its makeup. Ideal growing conditions for ginseng are humid summers with winter temperatures that dip below freezing, growing under a tree canopy, but there are variations even in places that meet this description. Several ginsenosides take five or six years to develop, and some even longer. According to scientific analysis, the optimum time to harvest ginseng root is when it is five to six years old. This is when the highest quantity of ginsenosides occurs, and when the root almost doubles in weight.[2]

Ginsenosides enter the blood about half an hour after taking ginseng. It takes about another hour and a half for tissues of the body to absorb them, at least according to animal studies. There is some question as to how much really gets into the blood when you eat ginseng. Only about one-fifth is absorbed when animals eat it and a large portion of this is excreted within six hours, apparently without being used. The amount of stomach acid and possibly other digestive conditions seem to affect absorption.

There is more to ginseng than ginsenosides. The root contains the antioxidant vitamins A, C and E, and selenium, germanium and maltol and ferulic acid. It also has the minerals calcium, magnesium, phosphorus and iron and traces of B1, B2, B12, pantothenic acid, niacin, folic acid, copper, iodine and zinc. These nutrients have several functions, including to fortify the body, fight off infection, and strengthen the nervous system. In addition, ginseng contains simple sugars, peptides and beta-sitosterol, which lowers cholesterol levels and reduces tumors.

The root is not the only part of the plant used medicinally. Flowers and leaves, which are much less expensive, are made into tea and added to baths in China. The tea is considered a good restorative, but it is seldom prescribed. According to herbal researcher and author Steven Foster, the folk tradition in the Ozark mountains of the southeastern U.S. uses the leaves as a tonic and to lower fevers. They contain active ginsenosides, but in different proportions than the roots. One assay found up to twice as many in the leaves.

🌿 THE MANY ROLES OF GINSENG 🌿

First and foremost, ginseng is an herbal adaptogen. What is an adaptogen? It improves general physical, mental and emotional health. An adaptogen does so by bringing numerous body functions into balance. It also helps you adapt to physical and emotional stress and to physical extremes, such as cold and hot or dark and light. Since ginseng improves physical and mental efficiency, you will find that it helps you work and think better and more efficiently.

The Russian scientist N. V. Lazarea coined the name "adaptogen" in 1947 to describe the action of several herbs he was studying. He decided that an adaptogen should meet three criteria. First, an adaptogen needs to normalize and balance various functions in the body. Second, its action should be nonspecific, meaning that it increases the entire body's general resistance to disorders or infections. Finally, it is safe to use, even over a long period of time. Ginseng easily meets all three of these criteria.

Ginseng's seemingly contradictory actions make it a difficult herb for scientists to pinpoint. Yet this is the very thing that makes ginseng so marvelous. Herbal researcher and author Dr. James Duke views an adaptogen such as ginseng as providing an "herbal potpourri" from which the body can select whatever action it needs to cure itself. This "potpourri" also makes ginseng a very safe herb to use. No wonder researchers get confused! Ginseng's adaptogenic approach differs from that of modern medicines, in which an individual compound has a single action.

In the course of doing its amazing balancing act in the body, ginseng plays opposite roles. A good example is its dual action on the central nervous system. It can be either a sedative or a stimulant. This action varies not only according to amount—large quantities tend to be more sedative and small ones more stimulating—but also from one person to the next. Likewise, ginseng lowers or raises blood sugar[3] and cholesterol. It protects red blood cells, but can also break them down, and it promotes or inhibits cell division. At the same time, it increases the cells' defense mechanisms. It inhibits or stimulates the heart and breathing rate, and regulates production of histamine. (Histamine dilates blood capillaries, constricts bronchioles, increases digestive juices in the stomach and can cause inflammation and headaches.) Ginseng quite possibly also influences sex hormones.

There are several other ways that ginseng normalizes bodily functions. It helps the liver process sugar and cholesterol and promotes their conversion into energy. Chinese studies have shown that ginseng oversees production of RNA, protein and DNA. RNA carries the cell's basic instruction plan and oversees protein synthesis. Long used to treat anemia in China, ginseng increases iron, red blood cells and protein in the blood.[4]

Another contribution to ginseng's adaptogen action is the several antioxidant compounds it contains (which are especially abundant in red ginseng). While oxygen is important to produce energy, it can also create havoc as it breaks down and makes harmful free radicals. These substances have an adverse effect on organs, causing cells to be destroyed, and they are now associated with promoting aging. Some researchers now say that oxidation is at least partially responsible for some liver disease, hardening of the arteries and degeneration of the eyes and nerves.

In looking at ginseng's variety of actions and trying to imagine how one herb can do so much, the logical assumption is that ginseng works through the body's own major regulators. The two areas of the brain that coordinate body activities are in the brain: the pituitary and the hypothalamus. If ginseng indeed taps into these glands, it gains influence over the entire body. The pituitary governs the body by regulating growth and the secretion of various hormones, including thyroid, adrenal and sex hormones. Due to its role in controlling hormones, it is sometimes designated as "the master gland," although this may better describe the hypothalamus.

Many of ginseng's effects on alleviating stress and fatigue, improving immunity and sexual functions, and maintaining blood pressure, blood sugar, water balance and body temperature are the very same actions controlled by the hypothalamus. This has led a few researchers to speculate that ginseng's primary action is on this gland. Like the pituitary, the hypothalamus plays several roles in the body and controls the release of hormones. It tells the pituitary what hormones to stimulate or to calm and also impacts hormones directly. It signals the adrenal glands when to pump adrenaline into the body in response to stress and when to shut it down. Basically the hypothalamus deals with whatever threatens the body's stability. This could be anything from a change in temperature or fatigue to a verbal attack or even emotional stress.

The core of many physical and emotional problems is stress. This might result in a number of seemingly unrelated problems. You acquire a chronic backache, get headaches, experience sugar cravings or sleep poorly. You may find your resistance is so low, you get almost every cold and flu that comes your way. Eventually, you feel tired all the time. Enjoyment may even drain out of life. Allergies, anemia, low blood pressure or weight loss may develop, making you feel more exhausted. Years of stress take a larger toll, possibly leading to heart disease, ulcers or mental confusion.

Stress itself is not the villain; what is important is how we to cope with it. The fortunate individuals who are able to handle stress creatively do better than those who carry the woes of the world on their shoulders. The problem is that while we still have the reflexes of a hunter or warrior, our adrenal alarm now goes off for much different reasons—we get caught in a traffic jam, the boss gets angry, the computer crashes, a family squabble ensues—all too often. Once vital for survival, these ancient responses are no longer always appropriate. When adrenal glands flood the body with adrenaline, nervous system action heightens, the heart pumps faster, blood rushes to your face, your eyes dilate and muscles flood with energy—all in a few seconds. You even begin to sweat in order to keep cool during the crisis.

Researchers find that people who have a tendency to be hostile pump out extra adrenaline every time they get upset. Then, once the crisis passes, they have difficulty calming down. As a result, they are more prone to high blood pressure and heart attack. A tool to help handle stress is to use an adaptogen such as ginseng. By simply reducing physical and emotional stress, ginseng should be able to help a large variety of problems. Ginseng even counters adrenal insufficiency, in which the overstressed glands shrink and can no longer perform properly.

Ginseng helps us deal with stress better by strengthening the adrenal glands. It also controls when they fire up and how quickly they shut down. One way it does this is by regulating a hormone called ACTH (adrenocorticotropic hormone), which stimulates adrenal activity. True to ginseng's adaptogen response, it regulates the level of ACTH and adrenaline depending upon the person who takes it. As a result, it normalizes people who are too hyped up and also those who are low on energy. Likewise, the amount of another adrenal hormone, hydrocortisone, can go up or down. In one study, it increased in the healthy volunteers and decreased in diabetics. Closely linked to the activity of cortisone, hydrocortisone regulates the body's metabolism of fats, carbohydrates, sodium, potassium and protein and decreases inflammation.

Yet, ginseng appears to be a selective stimulant. According to Dr. Shibata, the Japanese chemist who first named the ginsenosides, "In comparison with the effects of usual stimulants, the anti-fatigue action of ginseng shows an essential difference. The stimulants give effects under most situations, whereas ginseng reveals its action only under the challenge of stress." ACTH also influences moods by attaching itself to certain brain cells. The result is that you feel better and have more vitality.

The following sections discuss how ginseng specifically improves physical, mental and emotional stamina. They also tell of its ability to help heart conditions and enhance the immune system. Keep in mind while you read these that at the core of all these health improvements lie the adaptogenic qualities just discussed.

Physical Endurance

Physical fitness has become a way of life for millions of North Americans as they bounce, run, flex and prance their way to better health and bigger muscles. Vigorous yet prudent exercise, combined with diet, is their remedy for a flabby physique. However, some fitness addicts feel that exercise and diet are not enough to produce the body shape they want, so they turn to steroids—mostly the hormone testosterone—to bulk up muscles. The problem with steroids, however, is the side effects: they increase high blood pressure, nervous tension, headaches and nosebleeds, and produce skin and digestive problems. They can also result in a diminished sex drive and even sterility—a good example of what happens when you get too much of a good thing!

A better way to improve physical stamina is to turn to herbs, particularly ginseng. Ginseng's reputation for increasing stamina is more than 2,000 years old. In ancient China, two people—one with a piece of ginseng in his mouth and the other without—ran five li (a little less than two miles). If the runner chewing ginseng did not feel tired or out of breath at the end of this run, the root was considered genuine. In a modern version of this ancient study, one morning in 1948 Professor I. I. Brekhman gave Soviet soldiers ginseng before they ran a three kilometer race (again, a little less than two miles) and peeled off almost a minute from their average time.[5]

Ginseng is valuable to anyone who does physical labor and to both the professional and weekend athlete because it gives them the endurance they need to continue vigorous physical activity without tiring; they can go farther and faster. It improves endurance, respiration, oxygen consumption, muscle strength and the health of the cardiovascular system. The harder you walk, run, climb stairs or do any exercise, the more oxygen your body needs. Therefore, lung activity normally increases fairly quickly once muscles go into action to supply them with enough oxygen so they do not become fatigued. All that extra oxygen means less anaerobic (without oxygen) exercise that makes your pulse race, your heart pound, and your lungs strive to bring in more oxygen, causing you to pant trying to catch your breath. Such benefits to muscles and the cardiovascular system may not be immediately apparent, but studies indicate that ginseng's antifatigue properties are much more pronounced after it is used for at least two months. See the section on the heart and circulation (page 34) for a better understanding of how ginseng enhances oxygen utilization.

Ginseng improves physical energy in several other ways. One is by increasing the adrenal glands' production and secretion of corticosterone. This hormone in turn encourages the liver, muscles and other tissues to make and store glycogen from the carbohydrates we eat, then helps the body use it efficiently. When you need energy, glycogen breaks down into sugar and corticosterone controls its absorption into the cells. The hormone also regulates the cells' use of potassium and sodium, two minerals that work together to help cell metabolism by regulating fluids in the cells and maintaining a proper pH. Potassium balance is also essential for proper nerve impulses and muscle responses, especially in the heart.

There are other ways that ginseng helps physical strength and stamina. It encourages the production and storage of ATP (adenosine triphosphate), which is the enzyme that muscles store for fuel. Out of 150 herbs tested, ginseng stimulated ATP production the most. It may even contain a usable form of ATP.[6] Good physical stamina affects not only performance, but also how soon you recover after exercising—an important concern for the professional athlete who wants to build muscle, and for anyone trying to stay in shape. Of 30 people who took a ginseng product over several months, all but one found that it took them less time to recover after strenuous exercise. Not so in the placebo group, where only nine saw any improvement.[7]

Ginseng prevents overtaxed muscles from cramping and getting stiff and helps them recover quickly by reducing the amount of lactic acid in the blood. When muscles burn glycogen to get energy, they form lactic acid. Oxygen must be present to convert extra lactic acid back into glycogen to store for future use. If not converted, the lactic acid stays in the muscles and makes them cramp. In fact, one way that researchers gauge physical fatigue is to measure how much lactate, a salt derived from lactic acid, is in the blood. The less lactate there is, the better your endurance. When Drs. Ime Forgo and Gustav Schimert and colleagues at the Institute for the Prophylaxis of Circulatory Diseases at the University of Munich in Germany studied the effects of a standardized extract of ginseng on athletes for five years, they gave athletes ginseng and then measured their lactic acid levels before and after they exercised, the levels dropped. After nine weeks, the average lactate level was only half what it had been at the start of the experiment.[8] Ginseng's antioxidants also counter free radicals and other metabolic wastes responsible for causing oxidation that build up during strenuous exercise as muscle tissues break down.

Ginseng even provides some pain relief when muscles do become overworked and sore. It also helps prevent exhaustion from working or exercising in the heat. A popular traditional Chinese medicine tea blend includes ginseng to prevent overheating and to treat it if it does occur. When exercising or working in the heat begins to take its toll, the Chinese recommend combining ginseng and licorice (*Glycyrrhiza glabra*) with mulberry leaves (*Morus rubra*) and peony root (*Peony species*) to prevent heat exhaustion. Licorice root and schizandra berries (*Schisandra chinensis*) from China are other herbs that you can use with ginseng or Siberian ginseng to increase physical performance.

Siberian Ginseng

It is not surprising that millions of Russians greet each morning with a cup of Siberian ginseng tea. It has many of the same attributes as ginseng to improve stamina and endurance. Olympic-bound Russian athletes and cosmonauts find it helps them withstand environmental and physiological changes and maintain optimum health. On January 1, 1978, cosmonauts G. Grechko and J. Romanenko toasted in the New Year with a drink of Siberian ginseng. It also accompanied A. Ivanchenkov and V. Kovalenko on their record flight orbiting the Earth.

Like ginseng, Siberian ginseng improves your cardiovascular health and increases how much oxygen you inhale, absorb and use in your muscles. More oxygen gets to muscles to prevent anaerobic exercise that results in them cramping and getting stiff. It also ups the energy stored in muscles by almost one-third. The amount of glycogen produced from carbohydrates is also enhanced. In addition, Siberian ginseng helps overtaxed muscles recover more quickly and encourages muscle gain. In numerous studies, muscle tone, pulse rate and arterial blood pressure improved in the subjects and came back to normal faster than with a placebo.

Siberian ginseng was put to the test when Olympic athletes—including sprinters, high-jumpers, decathlon contestants, five- and ten-kilometer runners and marathon runners—found that they had better endurance and were willing to resume exercising sooner than usual when they took a tincture of Siberian ginseng before they went to sleep and one hour before they began training. On the other hand, members of a control group who did not take the herb were less active and took longer to recover. The Legraft Institute of Physical Culture and Sports also gave Siberian ginseng to competitive cyclists during the last 12 days of their races, and they captured six out of the ten first places. The cyclists noticed that they had more muscular vigor, their strength recovered sooner, they slept better and their appetites were better.[9]

To see how Siberian ginseng improved health under

difficult working conditions, it was given to seamen as a tonic while they were on a strenuous, two-month voyage in the tropics. Nearly three-quarters of the men did not experience the physical problems typical of doing hard work in such unfavorable conditions. Instead, their mental and physical capacity for work increased, and their heart function and breathing capacity improved. Siberian ginseng also maintained the seamen's balance of water to salt, blood protein and vitamin levels and kept their blood vessels in better shape.[10]

Mental Endurance

Accounts of herbs improving intelligence and memory were once regarded in the Western world as folklore. Now we know better; science is learning that ginseng can help the mind remain sharp, even as we grow older. While it is true that we normally become more forgetful as we age, only about one-tenth of North Americans over 65 have true senility and memory-loss disorders such as Alzheimer's disease. The good news, according to Stanford University psychiatrist Jerome Yesavage, M.D., is that most memory loss from age is reversible. A study funded by the National Institute on Aging followed people for 28 years and found that many showed no intellectual decline at all, even when they were well into their 70s. The study concluded that people turning 65 today are mentally sharper than previous generations, thanks to better nutrition and education. This is all the more reason to use ginseng to keep concentration, alertness and intelligence high. The idea is not new. The ancient Chinese herbal *Pen Tsao* recommended ginseng for "benefiting the understanding." Likewise, the Menomini Indians of the Great Lakes region regarded ginseng as a tonic to improve mental activity.

Unlike most stimulants, ginseng improves mental ability without disturbing sleep patterns, even when taken over a long period of time. Indeed, ginseng seems to be especially effective for people who notice a decline in their mental functions from age, illness or working under stress, not for those who are living a more healthy, balanced lifestyle. Ginseng helps in several arenas; it increases oxygen to the brain, provides more mental stamina and strengthens the adrenal glands so they can better counter the anxiety and stress that can clutter the brain channels. Studies from the Chinese Academy of Medical Science in Beijing, China showed that the ginsenosides in ginseng may also influence the activity of the brain by affecting neurotransmitters, chemicals that are released and controlled by the nervous system and influence many functions.

The brain needs plenty of oxygen to function properly. It demands one-fifth of the total oxygen carried in the blood. In fact, the most common cause of memory problems is hardening of the arteries, which slows blood flow to the brain. Several studies have examined how much ginseng can improve mental ability affected by circulation problems. One person interested in testing ginseng's ability to improve the brain's blood circulation is Italian researcher Dr. H. Quiroga. Two of his studies with capsules of a commercial ginseng extract prove good examples.

The people in one study did nothing else but take a ginseng tincture and the blood flow to their brain increased by an impressive 34 percent. In comparison, another group which took a placebo had almost no improvement. Although it is not quite as effective, researchers have compared ginseng's action to that of Hydergine, one of the most commonly prescribed drugs to treat problems that stem from poor brain circulation.[11] Even in elderly people whose circulation problems were moderate to severe, their arteries became more flexible and their brains and hearts received more blood with ginseng. In one study, improvement was considered "very favorable" in about one-third of nearly 200 people who were over the age of 40. Over 100 of these people experienced some beneficial results. The conclusion of the researchers from this and similar studies is that ginseng might be a good daily supplement for the elderly. They suggested that ginseng would be useful even in serious cases, if combined with drugs that protect blood vessels from degeneration.[12] Herbs that fit this description include ginkgo (*Ginkgo biloba*) and garlic (*Allium sativum*).

The following studies examine several different factors that are related to mental alertness: accuracy, concentration and coordination. On all of these accounts, ginseng made substantial improvement.

Several studies set up by Professor Brekhman in his Siberian lab during the 1960s looked at how much ginseng influences the mind, especially in accuracy. Brekhman chose radio and telegraph operators as his subjects because their jobs are stressful and demand quick decisions. The radio operators were asked to transmit messages for five minutes, which is almost twice the normal message length. Those who took ginseng increased their reading speed and could concentrate better than those who did not. The increase in their speed with ginseng was slight, but they made about half the number of mistakes as those who didn't take ginseng. The operators who did not get ginseng wore out and made 28 percent more mistakes. On the other hand, the ones who did get ginseng made 10 percent fewer mistakes.[13]

One researcher who read the results of Brekhman's studies was Professor Sandberg of Uppsala University in Sweden. They impressed him so much that he traveled to Russia and China to find out more about ginseng for himself. He returned to Sweden laden with ginseng samples and set up a series of elaborate, double-blind tests to test the psychomotor skills of students at the university. The tests involved tracing a complicated maze and crossing out randomly grouped letters. This same Swedish experiment had already been used to confirm coffee's stimulating effect on the mind. The students did equally as well as Brekhman's radio operators and proofreaders; they made about half the number of mistakes. Ginseng proved to have a stimulating effect much like coffee, but without creating the "jitters." As a result of these tests, Sweden's Health Ministry allowed ginseng products to bear declarations that they produced anti-fatigue effects.[14]

Professor Dörling of Hamburg, Germany studied the ability to concentrate. He measured this by seeing how quickly a person can discriminate between different light patterns. Dörling gave a strong dose of a commercial ginseng extract to 60 people for three months and gave another 60 a placebo. In the flicker-fusion test, they were asked to push a button the second they heard or saw an impulse. Eighty percent of the participants improved their speed with ginseng. In a similar experiment, they differentiated between changing light patterns. More than half the group taking ginseng could do so much faster. This was almost double the number of people who improved without ginseng. The ginseng group's reaction time remained faster even weeks after they stopped taking it. Although when they self-evaluated their improvement, they did not think that they were more alert, the tests showed that 10 percent of the ginseng group were. Even more significant, almost half of them had better concentration and memory.[15]

This same study also tested coordination. While hardly any improvement occurred with the people who got a placebo, there was a dramatic difference in the ginseng group. For some, their co-ordination improved almost immediately. After one month, ginseng was responsible for an improvement in over one-third of the participants. After another month, almost double that number had better coordination. By the study's end at three months, fully three-quarters were doing better, compared to only 16 percent in a placebo group.

Ginseng also influences the nerve growth factor, which helps rebuild nerve cells that relay messages from the brain throughout the body. Experiments by Japanese researcher Dr. H. Saito show that reflexes of the nervous system also improve. For example, after a person has been numbed under anesthesia, his nerve reflexes come back more quickly when he has taken ginseng beforehand.[16]

Siberian Ginseng

After Brekhman discovered Siberian ginseng's potential, he was eager to put it through the same tests that he had used with ginseng. Radio telegraph workers were again employed to test mental ability. As with ginseng, people in these studies increased their reading speed, concentration and accuracy and made far fewer mistakes. Several experiments later, it was concluded that Siberian ginseng can stimulate or depress nerve impulses in the brain. They determined that one way it improves work efficiency is through the central nervous system, and that people reach a mental response peak about eight hours after taking it. Brekhman described these and the following studies in his book, *Eleutherocrus Senticosus and Other Adaptogens Among the Far Eastern Plants*.[17]

Siberian ginseng also improves hearing and vision. Working with the Institute of Biologically Active Substances, Professor Stchichenkov did 60 tests to determine these effects on vision. He found that Siberian ginseng makes the eyes more responsive to light and able to see better in the dark. It also protects the ears from loud noises. The Institute is located by a seaport city, so it is not surprising that boat crew members were chosen for one of their research projects. Siberian ginseng was added to the crew's daily servings of stewed fruit. Even though these men were surrounded by loud and continual sounds while repairing their boat, they were better able to handle the noise. Their hearing tolerance improved by two to four decibels and they experienced less trauma to their inner ears than usual. The other half of the 39-man crew who received a placebo had no improvement. Brekhman concluded that Siberian ginseng directly reduces over-stimulation from loud noises in the hearing centers of the brain's cerebrum.

The memory of people who are senile or have mental disorders as a result of hardening of the arteries can also be expected to improve if they take Siberian ginseng for one to three months. This was true in one study even when the participants took a small amount of tincture: 5 to 20 drops daily a half-hour before each meal. In their program, they took it for one month, then had a ten-day break before resuming another round. Most of them reported that they could think much more clearly. As an added plus, they also felt stronger, some gained weight, and most felt more self-confident.

Emotional Stamina

Since the early 1950s, clinical studies have been done in Russia to demonstrate how ginseng helps people who suffer from nervous exhaustion and/or emotional problems. The best results occur when emotional disorders are related to nervous system problems. Ginseng also tends to help people with mood disturbances more than those who have psychoses, according to ginseng researcher and author, Stephen Fulder, Ph.D. It can reduce emotional distress, exhaustion, headaches, insomnia and uneasiness. Some people whose emotional problems cause them to be underweight find they develop a better appetite and put on more weight. As an added bonus, blood pressure is regulated and various symptoms of hormonal imbalance improve.

Fulder says that ginseng is widely used in Europe to treat depression, especially in the elderly. Italian researchers found that ginseng reduced depression and melancholy experienced by elderly subjects. It

also improved their general psychological performance, as well as their memory, and they had more
energy.[18] It also helps patients who feel unstable
emotionally, mentally dull, irritable, have low motivation and are generally indifferent to their sur-
roundings. In one study, some of the participants
had these symptoms and even more severe emotional problems. They were hostile, unsociable, un-
cooperative and they neglected their personal
hygiene. After using ginseng, their emotional state
improved significantly as well as their concentration and attention.[19]

A Chinese medical journal related the story of a
woman with adrenal deficiency who had undergone
much emotional stress in her life, including a very
hard pregnancy and labor. Instead of treating her
with the typical medical approach—cortisone and
ACTH, the pituitary hormone that stimulates the
adrenals into action—her doctors gave her licorice
root and ginseng to stimulate cortisone and ACTH
production in her body. The woman improved
quickly and the signs of adrenal exhaustion disappeared; she had more energy, gained weight and
her blood pressure returned to normal.[20]

Of course, you need not be emotionally disturbed
to seek stability from ginseng. British nurses in London who switched from day to night shifts found it
improved their competency as they struggled to ad-
just to their new routine. After three nights, most
nurses complained of disrupted sleep and fatigue, but
nurses who took ginseng were more alert, less emotional, more psychologically balanced and more tran-
quil than those not taking it. They also performed
better when tested for their coordination and speed.

Even though ginseng did not seem to improve their poor sleep, the nurses still felt slightly less tired. Ginseng also normalized blood sugar levels that had increased from the stress of the job change. Fulder, one author of this study, says, "The results, like virtually all these studies on ginseng, were not large, but they suggest some kind of improvement in stamina and competence in people who are pushed to their limit."[21]

One warning. If you already take a medication for emotional problems, be cautious about self-treating yourself with ginseng. It can reduce the effects of many sedatives and narcotics, probably in an attempt to bring the body back to a more harmonious balance.

Siberian Ginseng

When people suffering from various mental psychoses were treated for a month with Siberian ginseng, they were noticeably more cheerful, had more energy, and were much less irritable. When they continued the treatment for a longer period of time, most of them recovered. Their ability to do mental and physical work improved, and they slept and ate better. Some even gained weight. Everyone's health improved as well. They reported fewer headaches and other pains. Conditions normalized in those who had previously experienced heart weakness, palpitations or irregularity.

In a study with over 50 patients, aged 19 to 48, Siberian ginseng helped reduce their fatigue, insomnia, extreme exhaustion, irritability, feelings of unrest and problems keeping up with their usual work load.

They slept more soundly and their changed mental outlook produced a greater sense of well-being. The greatest improvements were seen in the people who previously had problems with exhaustion, feelings of inadequacy, depression, concentration, loss of appetite and insomnia.[22]

❀ HEART AND CIRCULATION ❀

Curious to discover how ginseng affects the cardio-vascular system, researchers found that it helps keep the heart at a healthy, low rate, while increasing the flow of blood to it. They speculate that taking ginseng as a mild heart tonic on a regular basis could reduce the number of deaths from heart attacks. The more forceful each contraction of the heart, the more blood it pumps, and the slower the heart needs to work. Athletes who took ginseng for nine weeks had a much lower heart rate during their maximum exercise than athletes given placebo pills. Ginseng's benefits even continue long after its use stops, with heart rates remaining low and improved lung action continuing for months.[23] Good heart performance and circulation are vital for physical, mental and emotional fitness. It takes a healthy, strong heart to circulate oxygen-rich blood through the body.

Ginseng is thought to work by regulating the heartbeat, selectively dilating arteries in the heart, and helping the heart muscle recover when it is injured due to lack of oxygen. It slows the heart rate, but at the same time, it increases blood flow. It also reduces the possibility of blood clots forming.

Tradition says sanchi ginseng (see the descriptions

of different ginseng species on page 7) normalizes the heart rate, blood pressure and circulation and helps prevent stress and fatigue. Its benefits for the heart are recorded in the *Pen Tsao Kang-mu,* and traditional Chinese medicine still prescribes it for these purposes.

Laboratory studies in China, as well as thousands of years of use there, have paved the way for Chinese hospitals to use herbs alongside Western drugs. The Wu-han Medical College and other hospitals in China now use sanchi ginseng to relieve the spasms and pain of angina. Studies at the college show it reduces symptoms in almost half of the people who take it. In one of these studies, all but one person had much less pain after taking ginseng.[24] The ginsenosides in this and other Panax ginsengs are excellent calcium channel blockers, which help to correct high blood pressure, angina pectoris and irregular heartbeat.[25] Chinese physicians often give the ginsenosides from ginseng to their patients after open heart surgery to decrease the chance of heart damage from lack of oxygen, and the patients who take it recover sooner. More willing than Western doctors to combine herbs with Western medicine, they also report excellent results combining ginseng with the heart medication digitalis to treat congestive heart failure. Red Ginseng increases digitalis's potency, so that lower doses of the drug are possible. This reduces the side effects that come from using the drug.[26]

Oxygen-Rich Blood

Ginseng also improves breathing in several ways that are important to physical and mental endurance, as well as general health. It increases the lungs' capacity to fill with air. Oxygen intake while resting has increased as much as 29 percent in only one month with daily doses of ginseng. Inhaling lots of oxygen-laden air is only part of ginseng's story. When you breathe, oxygen is drawn down into the lungs where tiny blood vessels absorb it, another function that ginseng helps. The oxygen-rich blood then circulates throughout the body, delivering oxygen to every cell. A person's true aerobic capacity is determined not by how much oxygen their lungs can hold, but by how much their body can absorb. Several studies done at the Institute for the Prophylaxis of Circulatory Diseases at the University of Munich in Germany show that ginseng increases oxygen absorption and utilization. Even after one nine-week study with athletes was over and they had stopped taking ginseng, their oxygen use was lower, but still remained well above average.[27]

Cholesterol

Cholesterol isn't all bad. After all, our bodies use it to make adrenal and sex hormones. However, when it clogs artery walls, it contributes to heart attacks. In 1984, the Coronary Primary Prevention Trial, a 10-year study in the U.S. of about 4,000 men, showed that lowering blood cholesterol reduces the risk of heart disease. While studying people who have high cholesterol at the Revitalization Center in Nassau, researcher Dr. I. M. Popov found that ginseng could drop cholesterol levels nearly 20 percent. The doctors of one 56-year-old man with a very high blood cholesterol level of over 325 had given him all the drugs they could to lower the level without success. After he took ginseng for only one month, his cholesterol dropped to almost normal. His high blood pressure followed suit and returned to normal as well.[28]

Sanchi ginseng is particularly successful at keeping down cholesterol. It increases the good type of cholesterol, HDL (high density lipoprotein cholesterol), which is thought to remove cholesterol plaque from the arteries. People who use ginseng over a long period of time tend to have lot of HDL in their blood, decreasing their chance of developing hardening of the arteries.[29] Ginseng also seems to make drugs that fight cholesterol work better.

Blood Pressure

If there is one good thing you can do for your health, it is to keep your blood pressure at a healthy level. When the effects of ginseng on human blood pressure are studied, it is found to produce varied results. Sometimes ginseng lowers and other times it increases blood pressure. It does this in part by increasing or decreasing the elasticity of the artery walls. Scientists conclude that small doses tend to increase blood pressure while large doses lower it, but that this action also depends upon the individual who takes it.

High blood pressure causes many problems, but most important, it increases the chances of dying from cardiovascular disease. Although drugs to treat high blood pressure are widely prescribed, they also have many side effects. According to long-term clinical studies from two 1985 issues of the *American*

Journal of Cardiology and the *Journal of the American Medical Association,* people who do not take medication are better off in the long run than those who do. As a result, doctors in Europe and Asia often prescribe herbs like ginseng before turning to drugs. In one study, a product containing both ginseng and ginkgo biloba, an herb widely prescribed in Europe for circulatory problems, dropped the systolic and diastolic blood pressure levels and increased blood flow in ten people with high blood pressure.[30]

There is controversy whether people with high blood pressure should take ginseng. The answer is that it is helps some people, but not others. Do not take chances with your health. Before treating blood pressure with any herb, discuss it with a knowledgeable health practitioner, especially if you are already taking medication. Other herbs that regulate blood pressure are hawthorn berries and flowers (*Crataegus oxyacantha*) and garlic (*Allium sativum*).

If low blood pressure is your problem, ginseng, especially American ginseng, can provide a much-needed mental and physical energy boost. American ginseng contains more of the ginsenoside (Rg) that affects blood pressure. Low blood pressure can be caused by several conditions, including infection, fever, anemia, excessive bleeding or a debilitating disease, and often results in fatigue. So little blood reaches the brain, simply rising from a chair may make the room start to spin. Chinese hospitals use ginseng to treat low blood pressure from shock.

Research at the Hwa-san Hospital in Shanghai found ginseng helped prevent heart attacks. It was given to patients who had irregular heart beats and an insufficient flow of blood to the heart which often precedes a heart attack. Ginseng brought their blood pressure back to normal, kept it there, and prevented them from going into shock. Patients who took ginseng recovered more quickly than those who did not. It turns out ginseng works even better than the pharmaceutical drugs that are typically given to such patients. While these drugs increase blood pressure, the effect is only temporary. The patients' blood pressures typically fall again in a short time, even when they are given repeated doses.

Siberian Ginseng

Like ginseng, Siberian ginseng normalizes blood pressure, raising or lowering it depending upon the person's need. In a series of studies conducted by the Soviet Academy of Sciences, it increased low blood pressure in over 50 patients who had rheumatic heart lesions. They were given only 20 drops of Siberian ginseng tincture three times a day for a month along with any conventional therapy they were already receiving. Other related effects that occurred were a better blood coagulation ability and more protein in the blood.

Siberian ginseng even helped speed recovery of patients from severe brain injuries they had received in accidents. When necessary, they were also treated with drugs, vitamins and surgery along with the Siberian ginseng. Compared to the placebo group, their blood pressure normalized faster, the circulation and blood vessel tone in their heads improved, and there were fewer irregularities in the muscles that line the heart (the myocardium). Nervous system disturbances associated with the heart and circulation, such as nerve signal transmission disturbances, blood vessel reflexes and inhibition signals were stabilized. Due to increased blood circulation in the brain, they were also able to perform much better on several mental tests.[31]

✣ IMMUNE ENHANCER ✣

General health is measured by the ability to fend off diseases, including the common cold, infections and allergies. As our understanding of immunity increases, so does the list of more serious immune-related diseases, among them psoriasis, asthma, multiple sclerosis, cancer, Epstein-Barr and chronic fatigue syndrome. Even arteriosclerosis and chronic infections like nephritis and colitis appear on the list. Immunity is also lowered by emotional or physical stress, poor diet (such as too many sweets), smoking and drinking too much alcohol. Even ''good'' stress, such as a vacation, can reduce the immune response.

Research indicates that ginseng improves our natural immunity. It increases the number of infection-fighting natural killer cells and white blood cells, as seen in a 1990 placebo study. When blood samples were analyzed for immune activity after one month, a whole range of positive changes had occurred in the ginseng group. Even greater improvement was seen after two months. Ginseng improved the activity of the immune system so much, the researchers conducting the study called the results ''drastic.''[32] While improving immunity and helping the body resist infection, ginseng also reduces pain, fatigue and fever.

One herbal formula used in both Japan and China to enhance immunity is Sho-saiko-to. This blend contains ginseng, along with several other herbs that include licorice (*Glycerriza glabra*), bupleurum (*Bupleurum falcatum*), and Chinese skullcap (*Scutellaria baicalensis*), an herb that stops certain viruses in their tracks and makes uninfected cells resist invasion. When the Mie University of Medicine in Tsu, Japan gave this formula to a group of healthy people, positive changes in immune activity that are responsible for destroying tumors were seen in their blood after one month. The combination of herbs worked better than any of the herbs alone.[33] Ginseng is often used with these immune-enhancing herbs, as well as astragalus root (*Astragalus membranaceus*), codonopsis root (*Codonopis pilosula*) and echinacea root (*Echinacea purpurea* and *E. angustifolia*).

Herpes

Several cases of herpes have successfully been treated with ginseng. One of these described in a scientific journal was a 66-year-old woman who had experienced occasional bouts for the last 10 years but recently began having outbreaks almost every month. After she took ginseng for a couple months, the blisters stopped appearing. She remained free of herpes even after she stopped taking ginseng. A 43-year-old man who had herpes for 27 years found that if he took ginseng regularly, no more outbreaks occurred. If he stopped, however, they came back with a vengeance.[34]

Cancer

When the National Cancer Institute investigated ginseng, it found no evidence that it helped cancer, although ginseng decreased tumor growth in at least one study with rats. Several Chinese herbal formulas traditionally used to treat cancer contain ginseng. One breast cancer formula combines ginseng with rhubarb (*Rheum species*) and ginger (*Zingiber officinale*). Modern Chinese doctors sometimes give ginseng to cancer patients while they undergo chemotherapy and radiation to lessen the side effects. If you consider doing this, consult a practitioner who is knowledgeable about herbs.

Some ginseng researchers consider it a better preventive than a cancer cure. Statistics from almost 2,000 individuals show that people who took ginseng on a regular basis did have fewer cancers of the mouth, lungs, stomach, liver, pancreas and ovaries. According to this survey, ginseng did not make any difference with cancer of the breast, cervix, bladder or thyroid. The most effective forms of ginseng were a fresh extract, white ginseng powder and red ginseng root. Fresh ginseng slices, a white ginseng tea and ginseng juice did not seem to decrease the risk of cancer.[35]

Siberian Ginseng

Siberian ginseng also enhances immune-system activity. Russian, German and American researchers independently discovered that it promotes production of interferon, which protects cells against viral infection. Siberian ginseng improves immunity by increasing the number of beta and alpha globulins in the blood. It also reduces excessive numbers of leukocytes in the blood. These scavenger cells move through blood and tissue fighting infection and high levels of them indicate that an infection is present.[36]

Siberian ginseng is often suggested for respiratory disease, especially to keep bronchial passages clear. Children treated for tuberculosis in a sanitarium at the Khabarovsk Medical Institute in Russia were given Siberian ginseng (one drop per year of age) for periods of 45 days with a two-week break in between. They also received additional therapies that included nutritional supplements and antibacterial drugs. Although they had been sick from two to four years, they improved considerably, especially when compared to a control group which was given only the non-herbal therapies. They could breathe better and did not get out of breath as easily as the other children; they were able to be much more physically active.[37]

The extremely cold working conditions in parts of Russia have offered the perfect test ground for Siberian ginseng. During the drastic temperature changes, workers always experience more colds, laryngitis, tonsillitis and sinus congestion. The incidence of colds and flu and related symptoms dropped 20 percent in over 1,000 Volzhsky factory test drivers who received Siberian ginseng in their thermos of tea every day, even though their work involved emotional and physical stress, as well as cold temperatures.[38] Sick days were cut almost in half for another 1,000 factory workers and nearly 500 healthy young men working in Siberia. The young men in Siberia also got a quarter of the usual number of sinus infections.

Dr. Khatiashvili of the Oncology Department of the Institute of Advanced Medical Training in

Tbilish, Russia gave Siberian ginseng for 14 days to 38 patients who were being treated for cancer with radiation. As a result, they had less nausea than a control group. They slept better, had a better appetite and did not have the usual breathing problems. Their tumors even healed more rapidly. The percentage of people who did not have their tumors return was larger in the group who took Siberian ginseng.[39] Over 400 elderly patients recovering from cancer-related operations had shorter hospital stays and felt less lethargy after the surgery with Siberian ginseng and vitamins, compared to 600 patients who did not take ginseng.

In Leningrad, the famous Petrov Oncological Institute found that cancer patients could tolerate 50 percent more of their drugs without side effects when they were given Siberian ginseng with the drug and surgery treatments. Those who got the Siberian ginseng and had surgery also lived an average of 17 months, five months more than patients who did not take it. Even the patients whose cancer had progressed so much that surgery was not an option survived for almost another year, more than twice as long as those who did not take Siberian ginseng.[40]

REPRODUCTIVE FUNCTIONS

Whether or not ginseng affects hormones is a question that has puzzled researchers for some time. According to history, it does. Traditional Chinese medicine tells us that ginseng "strengthens exhausted sperm and impotent genitals." It also has a long reputation of being an aphrodisiac. For thousands of years, Chinese folklore told stories of how ginseng improves virility, as well as stamina and longevity. That is one reason Chinese herbalists still recommend it for men and women over 40. In North America, Indians used ginseng to promote fertility for both men and women. The Delaware and Mohegan tribes recommended it for numerous afflictions of the sexual organs and the Cherokee believed it strengthened the womb.

However, studies claiming that ginseng contains hormones have not been supported. To date, people do not show any changes in their hormones after they take ginseng. The people who have been tested were all healthy, so perhaps they did not need their hormones changed. Chances are that if ginseng does affect hormones, it does so by stimulating the brain's hypothalamus and pituitary to alter production of sex hormones and possibly by making certain cells more or less receptive to hormones.

Many of ginseng's properties appear to be related to the hormonal system. Unfortunately, we know far more about how ginseng affects the sex life of animals than people! It does increase sex hormones in rats and rabbits and is a uterine toner, but only in very high doses. It also increases the male hormone testosterone and increases the weight of the sex organs in male and female rats; the males have more sex when they are given ginseng. It also increases prolactin, which in turn boosts progesterone[41] and seems to discourage estradiol, a potent and possibly carcinogenic form of estrogen.

Chinese herbalists have recommended ginseng for pregnant women for centuries to give them extra energy. When nearly 100 pregnant women took ginseng in one study, they had less pre-eclampsia, a type of toxicity that can occur during pregnancy, than women who took no ginseng.[42] However, in case ginseng does have hormonal action, be cautious about using it during pregnancy and do not do so unless it is advised by an herbalist or doctor.

Menopause

Ginseng does relieve many menopausal complaints, and this has been backed by several studies with large groups of women. In one German study, over half of the 72 menopausal women given ginseng found that all their symptoms—hot flashes, night sweats, nervous tension, headaches and heart palpitations—completely disappeared when they took ginseng. In comparison, this was true for only 19 percent of the placebo group. The women experienced less depression and insomnia and fewer sexual problems. R. T. Owen, M.D., the gynecologist who did this study suggests that women should take ginseng well before menopause begins to prevent the symptoms from even starting. She also adds, "If they receive this safe geriatric treatment regularly over a longer time, they will not require hormones."[43]

Ginseng is especially effective for hot flashes, and often completely eliminates them within six weeks. Dr. Robert Atkins, M.D., a well-known author and doctor of nutritional medicine, agrees. He found that out of hundreds of patients who complained about having hot flashes, about 80 percent of them responded to ginseng. The few women who do not get results from ginseng do so once they add vitamin E to their regime. Many herbalists have noticed that vitamin E does seem to enhance actions of herbs such as ginseng.

Other herbs for women to take with ginseng for menopausal symptoms are black cohosh root (*Cimicifuga rasemosa*), vitex berry (*Vitex agnus castus*), licorice root (*Glycyrrhiza glabra*), dong quai root (*Angelica sinensis*), motherwort leaves (*Leonorus cardiaca*) and fenugreek seed (*Trigonella foenumgraecum*).

Impotence and Male Menopause

Several Chinese folk tales tell of men in their 90s fathering children after taking ginseng. As far as we know, these are only stories, but if any herb inspires passion and maintains fertility, ginseng is a good candidate. Clinical studies from Japan, Russia and the Chinese Medical Research Institute indicate that ginseng can help male impotence when it is caused by physical problems. Japanese and Korean hospitals have been using ginseng extracts for decades to treat impotence and also some sexual problems in women.[44]

In studies quoted by the Ginseng Research Institute, it was concluded that ginseng indirectly helps men who do not have sufficient sex hormones. Several studies done in China indicate that ginseng increases the sperm's mobility and raises the sperm count in men who have low numbers. Other herbs to consider combining with ginseng to help eliminate impotence are yohimbe bark (*Pausinystalia yohimbe*), wild oats (*Avena sativum*), ginkgo (*Ginkgo biloba*) and perhaps damiana leaves (*Turnea aphrodisiaca*).

Although men don't participate in obvious hormonal cycles like women, researchers speculate that they do have a male cycle and also experience male menopause. Symptoms of male menopause are similar to those experienced by women during menopause—irritability, anxiousness, fatigue and decreased ambition, and sometimes even hot flashes and night sweats. When male menopause hits, ginseng can strengthen the adrenal glands, increase physical and mental stamina and decrease the stress hormones that can lower testosterone levels.

Siberian Ginseng

Professor Brekhman considered Siberian ginseng an even stronger sexual stimulant than ginseng and called its action gonadotropic, or one that stimulates the function of the gonads (sex glands). It is used extensively in the Soviet Union to stimulate breeding in animals, where its benefits have been observed mostly in animals with retarded growth or poor development.

✤ OTHER CONDITIONS TREATED BY GINSENG ✤

Blood Sugar Control

Ginseng's ability to help diabetics was probably recognized as early as the first century A.D. when the *Ming-I-Pieh-lu* described how it reduces excessive thirst, fatigue and excessive urination—common symptoms of the disease. In diabetes, blood sugar levels are elevated due to an insufficient amount of insulin. Several of the compounds in ginseng increase insulin in the blood. Before insulin was available in the 1920s, Japanese hospitals treated diabetic patients with ginseng, to successfully reduce their blood sugar levels and symptoms. In dozens of clinical studies, ginseng also eliminated symptoms of diabetes, especially the excessive thirst and also impotence. Most diabetics also feel less tired when they take it. Several studies from China show that ginseng lowers blood sugar levels of diabetics from 40 to 50 percent, and even returns some levels to normal. And these levels remain low for a week or two after the ginseng is discontinued.

Diabetics who are resistant to insulin have been able to reduce the amount they take with ginseng. In a study involving 21 patients who have diabetes mellitus, more than half of them improved after they started taking large daily doses (2700 mg) of Korean red ginseng. In about two months, blood sugar levels of the type II diabetics who were not taking insulin also dropped. In one study, their body weight increased and their moods and motivation improved as well. No one reported any side effects.[45]

Researchers at Japan's Sanraku Hospital in Tokyo and The Osaka University School of Medicine in Osaka saw impressive results when they gave diabetics capsules of ginseng with vitamin E. This combination successfully treated complications from diabetes that were caused by poor circulation, such as nerve and kidney damage, impaired function of the retina and impotence. It also helped them feel less tired. It was determined that 600 mg a day of ginseng may be necessary at the beginning of the treatment, then the dosage can be dropped by half for continued therapy.[46]

If you are a diabetic on insulin, be careful when taking anything that may alter your blood sugar. Ginseng is not a reliable replacement for insulin so consult with a medical practitioner knowledgeable about herbs and be sure to check your blood sugar regularly.

Siberian Ginseng

In Russia, Siberian ginseng has been used extensively to treat diabetes because it stabilizes blood sugar and alleviates depression and fatigue. Even healthy subjects who drank sugar water experienced almost no rise in their blood sugar, even during the first hour. Instead, blood sugar was slightly below its initial level by the end of the third hour. One Russian researcher suggested that Siberian ginseng could successfully treat mild forms of diabetes, and also recommended it be used with insulin for more severe cases.[47]

Liver Damage and Kidney Stones

Ginseng counteracts the toxic effects of drugs like amphetamines and poison such as chloroform. European research shows that ginseng even slightly improves chronic liver disease in elderly patients whose livers have been injured by too much alcohol or too many drugs. After they started taking ginseng, their liver enzyme counts improved, even though their livers were already quite damaged.[48]

People recover more rapidly from alcohol's effects, even a drunk stupor, with ginseng. According to preliminary studies, ginseng encourages detoxification by stimulating two liver enzymes, alcohol dehydrogenase and aldehyde dehydrogenase, which are responsible for converting alcohol in the liver to a less toxic form. When healthy volunteers drank too much alcohol, four drinks (2.5 ounces of 50 proof vodka for every 140 pounds of body weight) in 45 minutes, ginseng kept their blood alcohol much lower than when the same men drank alcohol without ginseng. Seventy percent had up to half the amount of alcohol in their blood.[49]

Ginseng has been compared to allopurinol, a drug that strongly inhibits the uric acid that commonly forms kidney stones and occurs in excessive amounts in people who have gout.

Rheumatoid Arthritis

The Chinese use ginseng to treat rheumatoid arthritis, which makes joints stiff and painful, because it stimulates production of adrenal hormones like hydrocortisone that reduce inflammation. Instead of the adverse side effects caused by prescription drugs like prednisone, ginseng has an opposite action. While the drugs eventually shrink the size of adrenal glands and impair their function, ginseng reverses adrenal shrinkage. Ginseng offers another benefit to arthritics by enhancing their immune systems. Other antiarthritic Oriental herbs often used with ginseng to reduce inflammation are the roots of bupleurum (*Bupleurum falcatum*), licorice (*Glycyrrhiza glabra*) and turmeric (*Curcuma longa*). Western herbs include the roots of echinacea (*Echinacea species*) and yucca (*Yucca species*).

Skin Care

One unique use of ginseng is as a cosmetic. When applied to the skin in a moisturizing face cream, ginseng seems to be an antiaging agent that regenerates the skin and reduces wrinkles.[50] Ginseng creams also improve acne conditions and reduce severe itching of the skin. For years, ginseng has been added to some expensive facial creams. At least one new skin lotion contains ginseng with vitamin E and aloe vera.

Siberian Ginseng

The dermatology clinic of the Vladivostok medical clinic found that Siberian ginseng treats several skin diseases. It slows down baldness that is associated with excessive production of sebum, the scalp's oil. Scalp inflammations and dandruff gradually disappeared completely in all the 100 people participating in one study. They applied a lotion containing Siberian ginseng on their scalps and also drank a Siberian ginseng extract. The oil production of their scalps normalized and their hair stopped falling out. They even reported an extra benefit: their mood improved!

✤ WHO SHOULD TAKE GINSENG: HOW MUCH, HOW LONG? ✤

Ginseng is probably sold in more forms than any other herb. Like most herbs, it is available as a tea, tincture or in capsules (generally 300 to 500 mg). Tinctures and other types of extracts may also be dehydrated and made into capsules or tablets. Tinctures work the fastest, since the various components in ginseng have already been partially broken down in the tincture-making process, although fast action is not necessarily required in a tonic.

A generic dose is one to three pills, a few cups of tea or one to three dropperfuls of tincture daily. Since ginseng is such a popular herb, many teas, tinctures and pills use it as part of a formula, blended with other herbs and sometimes nutritional supplements. In most cases, you would take the same amount of formula as suggested for ginseng alone. However, it is difficult to generalize about the wide spectrum of ginseng products available. The best time to take ginseng is between meals, although there are always exceptions depending upon the person and his or her condition.

To make a tea, bring a teaspoon of sliced or powdered ginseng root per cup to a boil in a pan of water. Simmer very gently for 20 to 30 minutes, take off the heat and let steep for at least another 20 minutes. Strain out the ginseng and it is ready to drink. It will store in the refrigerator if you wish to make a large enough amount to last for a few days. Generally, the roots can be resimmered, although the second batch of tea will not be as strong as the first. If you want to make whole roots into tea, break off a piece and soak it overnight so it will be soft enough to cut.

You can purchase a ginseng cooker in a Chinese herb store and some Chinese variety stores if you would like to brew your tea in the traditional manner. These cookers are a porcelain or sometimes a clay double boiler in which you can prepare any type of herb tea. The taste of ginseng by itself does not appeal to most people, so you may want to add a pinch of some tastier herb to the tea, such as ginger powder or a few slices of fresh ginger root from the grocery store.

A small piece of the ginseng root can also be bitten and chewed. In addition, you can find ginseng sold in small vials that contain a diluted and sweetened extract of ginseng or ginseng combined with bee pollen or other herbs. Each of these vials is one dose. Similar ginseng elixirs come in larger bottles as well. Since extracts and elixirs vary in strength, follow the dose recommended on the product. There also are ginseng sodas, candies, toffees, even ice cream and chewing gum! Dosage is not a consideration with these products. They usually do not contain much ginseng, but may have enough for a slight pick-me-up.

Your general health, constitution and the condition for which you are taking ginseng all influence the appropriate dose. It is best to stay with small doses unless you are working with a health care practitioner who suggests a larger amount. The typical recommendation is to take a quarter to a half a gram of ginseng twice a day, two hours before a meal. That is up to one gram a day. Most North Americans do not think in terms of grams, but rather of ounces, but grams are an easier measurement when discussing such small amounts. (One ounce by weight is slightly more than 30 grams.) If you buy prepackaged ginseng the number of grams or ounces should be indicated on the label. It is better not to take ginseng after an evening meal since this can be too stimulating. Continue taking it for four to six weeks, followed by a two- to four-week interval. In some cases, people prefer to take ginseng continuously, especially the chronically ill or elderly.

A popular new way to sell ginseng is as "standardized" extracts. This guarantees that the product contains a certain amount of ginsenosides. The French *Pharmacopoeia* requires ginseng products to have at least 2 percent ginsenosides to be officially recognized, and both Germany and Switzerland require a minimum of 1.5 percent. Ginsenosides are compounds in ginseng that science has determined are the active ingredients. To understand more about them, read the section on ginseng's chemistry and pharmacology (page 11).

While being able to offer a standardized product is considered a guarantee that the product is superior, there are several pros and cons to standardization. One advantage is obvious. It is difficult for the consumer to tell if ginseng has been adulterated or is of poor quality. In Taiwan, researchers tested 37 samples of commercial ginseng off the shelves of stores. They found that the amount of ginsenosides varied considerably from one product to the next and some even contained other herbs instead of ginseng.[52]

Many medical doctors feel more comfortable with standardized herbs because they know the percentage of "medicine" in them. This makes herbs seem more comparable to the drugs that they commonly use. At first, this may seem an advantage and in some regards it is. It means that more physicians will be interested in using herbs. However, in focusing on a single standardized compound, we should not forget the rest of the herb. One beauty of herbalism is how the integrated compounds in a plant work together.

This concept is lost when one compound is extracted from an herb to produce a drug and may also be lost in the frenzy to standardize herbs.

Standardization does assure that a product is ginseng and that it contains the active ingredient, although it does not necessarily guarantee that it is good quality. Standardization is only as good as the particular standards a company uses. In other words, standardization itself is currently not standardized, so one company's 1.5 percent could be another company's 3 percent.

Ginseng keeps quite a while. As with other herbs, the best way to store it is in the whole form, rather than cut or powdered. Also keep it in a dry, airtight container, since exposure to moisture breaks down the major compounds much faster. Ginsenosides are fairly stable, but do break down with age. When ginseng was tested after being stored for three years, there was 27 percent less of these compounds in the white root and 12 percent less in red ginseng.[53]

🌿 CONTRAINDICATIONS 🌿

Studies on ginseng report that it is very safe and has few side effects. Herbal researcher and author Dr. James Duke considers the ginsenosides found in ginseng about 10 times less toxic than the caffeine from coffee and black tea or the theobromine found in chocolate.

There are a few cautions for taking ginseng. It can increase blood pressure and lower blood sugar so if you have high blood pressure or diabetes, consult with a health practitioner knowledgeable about herbs before taking it. Ginseng may also be too stimulating for many people who are manic or schizophrenic or simply very nervous. Be especially cautious about ginseng if you take antipsychotic drugs. Ginseng also may not mix well with other pharmaceutical drugs since it some-times delays their absorption, at least in test animals. There is a possibility that it could also alter hormonal treatments. It is better not to mix it with stimulants like coffee because it can over-stimulate the body.

Depression and nervous system problems have been reported in China with people who took ex-tremely large quantities—around 50 grams a day, or over 50 times the recommended daily dose. Most scientific studies use large amounts, usually three to nine grams a day. Taking more than that is not a good idea. Anyway, even large amounts such as 10 grams are not absorbed by the body as well as smaller amounts.[52] Other possible side effects from taking lots of ginseng, usually for an extended time, are heart pain and palpitations, vomiting, earaches, nosebleeds, a decrease in sexual potency, headaches, itchy skin eruptions, diarrhea and low white blood cell count.

✿ MISLABELING AND ADULTERATION ✿

Ginseng has endured several controversies over its safety. The most publicized was the 1979 Siegal Report. It reported that the root overstimulated the central ner-vous system, resulting in depression, nervousness and high blood pressure.[54] The media, quick to pick up a negative story on a popular herb, blew the study's data out of proportion. Even today, some people are still leery about ginseng because they vaguely remember these newspaper stories. What the news reports failed to mention is that unusually large amounts of ginseng, described as "recreational doses," were used and that these were often taken along with lots of coffee and sometimes drugs that can increase ginseng's stimulating action.

Ginseng was again subjected to media attack in 1990. This turned out to be a case of mislabeling. A Canadian baby was born with excessive body hair, a hormonal problem probably due to too much of the sex hormone testosterone in his mother's blood. She had been drinking a tea mistakenly labeled "Siberian ginseng." Both Siberian ginseng and ginseng itself were quickly accused of causing birth defects in a flurry of negative newspaper stories as reporters confused the two herbs. It took awhile for the dust to settle, but Denis Awang, Ph.D., then chairman of Canada's Health Protection Branch of Health and Welfare, determined that the herb tea was really Chinese silk vine (*Periploca sepium*), an herb sometimes sold as Siberian ginseng. It was eventually determined that even this herb had nothing to do with the baby's condition. However, years later, rumors and fear over ginseng's use continue.[55]

Like all expensive or popular herbs, ginseng is subject to adulteration. Throughout history, sly merchants have substituted other roots in its place. Plants like ginseng used to be traded in their whole form to assure the buyer was getting the right merchandise and good quality. In this age of packaging, ginseng is often sold as liquid tinctures or in capsules, making it difficult to determine its quality, or combined with other herbs so it's often hard to know what you are getting.

Unfortunately, mislabeling is a problem with both ginseng and Siberian ginseng. It does not help that the Chinese silk vine has the same common Chinese name as Siberian ginseng, *wu-jia-pi,* meaning "five-leaf, spiny bark." Apparently the confusion goes back hundreds of years. In the eleventh century A.D., Su Song tried to sort it out in his *Tu Jing Pen Tsao (Illustrated Herbs).* Today, Siberian ginseng is supposedly called *ci-wu-jia* while the silk vine is designated as *xiang-jia-pi,* although silk vine is still sold as Siberian ginseng and problems with mislabeling continue. In 1987, when the American Herb Association had an independent lab analyze five different products labeled Siberian ginseng with chromatography and microscopic identification, only two proved to be the real thing. The others were apparently Chinese silk vine.

Probably the most outlandish marketing story is that of "wild red desert ginseng." More accurately named canaigre or tanner's dock (*Rumex hymenosepalus*), this is a relative of yellow dock with similar properties. High in tannins, it is an astringent used to ease diarrhea and sore throats. The company selling it described a "new" herb that was created when ginseng seeds fell out of the pockets of 19th century Chinese laborers working on the railroad in the Southwest U.S. The seeds supposedly germinated and managed to survive in the desert just long enough to flower and cross-pollinate with dock, thus creating a plant that looks like dock, but with all the properties of ginseng. Eventually, the American Herb Products

Association cracked down on this botanical impossibility and convinced the company to change their labeling.

❧ AN ENDANGERED PLANT ❧

Few of the early 'shang traders probably considered the impact that collecting millions of tons of wild ginseng made on the American wilderness. To them, ginseng must have seemed an abundant resource, so they filled their bags with roots and their pockets with money as they depleted the woods of plants. In the 1770s, North America was exporting an average of 140,000 tons of ginseng roots every year. One 1773 shipment alone from Boston weighed 55 tons! The year 1824 set a new record, at over 600,000 tons of roots.

Unfortunately, while they learned from the Indians to identify the plant, the ginseng harvesters did not adopt careful harvesting practices like those of the Ojibwa, who lived around Lake Superior. The Indians were careful to harvest the roots only after ginseng's berries had turned red, when they contained seed. The seeds were planted back into the hole where they dug the root to assure another plant would replace the one taken. Today, ginseng is considered threatened or endangered in four states: Kentucky, Tennessee, Virginia and Illinois. It is illegal to wildcraft ginseng in many states without a permit and most states restrict digging wild ginseng, except from August to November. However, these regulations are not always respected. The Convention on International Trade in Endangered Species (CITES), the

U.S. Fish and Wildlife Service, and the Department of Agriculture regulate the ginseng trade. A federal permit is required to export either farm-grown or wild American ginseng. Even so, more than 14,500 pounds of wild American ginseng roots were exported to Asia in 1992.[56]

With prices topping $600 a pound for wild American ginseng, it is no wonder people still dig it. One solution is for consumers to buy only farm-cultivated ginseng or "woodsgrown" ginseng, grown under a natural tree canopy of hardwood forest with as few pesticides as possible. Unfortunately, ginseng is a vulnerable crop and farmers tend to use many pesticides and herbicides.

China also grows woodsgrown ginseng, a root that rarely reaches the U.S. When it does, it can sell for thousands of dollars per ounce. Wild Korean ginseng is even more expensive, going for around $20,000 an ounce in the U.S. when available. With the long history of use in China, wild ginseng is even less abundant there than in North America.

THE CHINESE VIEW OF GINSENG

Traditional Chinese medicine uses a complex system to identify an herb's properties and identifies these by describing its "energetics," such as heating, cooling, expanding or contracting. It also looks at the ability of herbs to direct or move chi, the body's vital life force. Ginseng is regarded as a general tonic with a combination of sweet and bitter with warming characteristics. As a tonic, ginseng is found in many formulas that strengthen weak conditions, such as general fatigue or weakness, anemia, lack of appetite, shortness of breath, nervous agitation, forgetfulness, thirst and impotence. While it is rarely used by itself in Chinese medicine to treat specific disorders, it is often combined with other herbs to enhance many different types of treatments. As a result, out of nearly 500 Oriental prescriptions that were surveyed, over a quarter contained ginseng.

Different forms of preparation are important to Chinese medicine, not because of the attractiveness of the presentation, but because according to its principles, they change the energy of the plant. As a result, great care goes into the slicing and packaging of an herb.

Not only are various characteristics of an herb considered, but so is a patient's constitution. Categorizing the herb and the person helps the Chinese practitioner determine which herb is most appropriate for an individual. The result is a system of medicine that is much more individualized than Western medicine as well as one that is very foreign to Western-trained practitioners. While these concepts can be interpreted into Western medical terminology to some degree, much is lost in the translation.

From a traditional Chinese medicine perspective, ginseng is incompatible with certain conditions or individuals. For example, it is considered warming, so it is generally not given to someone who has a fever or an infection. Another example of someone who may have too much heat is a person who is hot-tempered, physically strong and has a strong sexual drive. They may find taking ginseng a "burn-out." Typically, a healthy, energetic person under 40 need not take ginseng unless he or she is under physical or emotional stress. An old Chinese saying goes, "What will a person take when they are old if they take ginseng when they are young?" Rather than try to explain Chinese medicine here, these concerns are better addressed by an acupuncturist or other herbal practitioner who works in the Chinese system.

Westerners who believe Oriental ginseng is superior to American ginseng are misinformed. The Chinese who buy enormous quantities of American ginseng certainly do not feel this way. More accurately, they actually regard American ginseng as a different herb. In Chinese terms, it raises less heat in the circulatory, respiratory and digestive systems (and is therefore less "yang"). This makes American ginseng a popular tonic in hot tropical and subtropical regions of Asia. It can also be given to someone who has a fever.

Perhaps the notion comes from the fact that ginseng root looks like a man, but the popular rumor that **gin**seng is not for women, but only for men is also not true. Oriental diagnostics is much more concerned with the constitution of an individual, not in his or her sex. In fact, ginseng is common in formulas for women during menopause.

❧ GRADING AND PROCESSING GINSENG ❧

According to the traditional Chinese system of medicine, the quality of a ginseng root is determined by many factors. These include its age, shape, size, overall condition and where it was grown. Most quality roots are harvested when they are six to twelve years old. This can be determined by counting the ridgelike scars on the neck—one for each year. For the root to be considered a good grade, this "neck" section on top of the root must be present. Most roots are sold when they are about six years old and from four to five inches long. The Koreans name their ginseng roots Heaven, Earth, Good and Tails. "Tails" refer to the long, narrow rootlets at the bottom, and these are the least potent and the cheapest.

Of course, the better the root's quality, the higher the price. Ginseng claims the distinction of not only being the most popular herb sold, but also one of the most expensive. The price of cultivated white Korean ginseng roots ranges from $80 to $200 a pound depending upon the quality. It is also possible to pay hundreds of dollars for just one root of exceptional quality. American ginseng is not graded and currently sells for around $50 to $100 per pound. There is also an American red ginseng that is prepared with a process similar to the one used to make Oriental red ginseng. It is a little more expensive than white American ginseng.

China White

A new category, white ginseng is grown in China from imported North American ginseng seeds. It is currently being sold at low (for ginseng) prices. It sells for less than $60 a pound to test the market for it. Unscrupulous dealers sometimes mix the less expensive China white with American-grown ginseng to make an extra profit since it is difficult to tell the difference.

Red Ginseng

A popular way to process ginseng is to steam the unpeeled, fresh roots with herbs such as red and white peony root, cinnamon and dates. The roots may be first soaked in honey or wine. The result is a deeply colored red root that is somewhat hard and brittle. Since only high-quality roots are processed and the process itself is thought to enhance the root's medicine, red roots are considered superior to white roots. They are also considerably more expensive. When analyzed, red ginseng contains the same major ginsenosides as white ginseng, but also has four additional ginsenosides. The red Korean roots are more valuable than red roots from China.

Red ginseng is so stimulating that it is used with more caution than unprocessed white ginseng. It is common to recommend it to people who are over 40 years old and have strong constitutions, although the Chinese sometimes prescribe it to the weak and debilitated to increase their strength. Korea controls red and white ginseng through their Office of Monopoly. Before white roots are allowed out of the country, their outer, pale brown skin is removed to expose the white root. Peeling them prevents processing them into red ginseng in another country. It also makes the white roots inferior from a chemical point of view since the skin contains most of the ginsenosides.

Red roots are sold by the caddy and graded from 1 to 6, with 1 being the largest and most superior. A caddy equals 600 grams, slightly more than 1¼ pounds. Ginseng prices fluctuate, but you can expect to pay from $85 to $180 a pound for red ginseng.

🌿 OTHER "GINSENGS" 🌿

Several other herbs also bear the name ginseng. Most
are not well known in North America and have been
labeled "ginseng" because they also have adaptogenic properties. These herbs, however, can be considered direct substitutes for ginseng, but should be
regarded on their own merits.

FALSE GINSENG: CODONOPSIS (*Codonopsis pilosula*)

Codonopsis is considered a milder and less stimulating version of ginseng in China, where it is called
dang shen. Another name is "poor man's ginseng"
because it is much cheaper than ginseng, although
almost twice as much of it is generally used. It is
often regarded as an even better toner for the spleen
and lungs than ginseng itself. It is used to treat fatigue, appetite loss, diarrhea and bronchitis and to
prevent stomach ulcers. Chinese doctors regularly
give it to heart patients to reduce blood clots. It enhances immunity and counters the adverse effects of
radiation treatments. A sweet-tasting root, it is a common ingredient in Chinese medicinal soups.

PRINCE'S GINSENG (*Pseudostellaria heterophylla*)

A general tonic in China, this member of the carna-
tion family is common in China and much less expensive than true ginseng. Unlike ginseng, it is not
a true adaptogen, but does help restore energy and
assist digestion and food assimilation. It is recommended for increasing strength and appetite during
and after a chronic illness. Animal studies indicate

that it enhances the immune system by stimulating natural killer cells and T-cells and decreasing the size of cancerous tumors.

WOMEN'S GINSENG: DONG QUAI (*Angelica sinensis* or *S. acutiloba* in Japan)

Dong quai, also spelled *dang gui* and *tang kwai,* is currently popular in North America for easing menopausal symptoms and regulating menstrual cycle problems, such as painful, irregular or scanty periods. It also has a long reputation for promoting fertility in women and approximately a half billion Chinese women use it as a daily tonic, often adding it to soups and stews. The Chinese say it builds up the blood and give it to women whose energy is depleted. It has not been proven to influence hormones, although it can either stimulate or relax the uterus. It also improves the health of the liver and is used to treat liver diseases, such as hepatitis and cirrhosis. Like ginseng, it is good for the heart and circulation, increasing blood flow through the heart, improving utilization of oxygen and helping prevent blood clots and hardening of the arteries. It also seems to encourage development of red blood cells. In addition, dong quai reduces inflammation, is antibiotic and is a mild sedative. Since it increases menstrual bleeding, it can be a problem if used when a woman has fibroids or endometriosis. Also, it should not be taken without professional supervision with pharmaceutical drugs, especially blood-thinners or heart medication, or when there is a chronic illness.

CALIFORNIA GINSENG: CALIFORNIA SPIKE-NARD (Aralia Californica)

A member of the Aralia or ginseng family, and related to the spikenards of the eastern U.S. California spikenard grows up to 10 feet high, looking like a giant ginseng. Its root crown also bears scars of each year's growth. The spikenards were greatly valued by the Native Americans to treat numerous complaints and all of them have been suspected of having at least some properties that are similar to ginseng. Several spikenards, including Aralia racemosa of both eastern North America and Asia, were used as digestives and women's tonics and to treat asthma and blood poisoning. As far as we know, California spikenard was primarily for lung problems and the root was chewed during long hikes to prevent thirst and increase energy. The root was also used during a debilitating disease or a viral infection like herpes, and applied externally to rashes.

OREGON GINSENG: DEVIL'S CLUB (Opopanax horridum)

A member of the Aralia, or ginseng family, devil's club got its name from the threatening-looking spines that cover its large stems and fan-shaped leaves. Some herbalists suspect that this native of the Pacific Northwest is an adaptogen. Native Americans used the stem and root bark to treat general sickness, pain, rheumatism and lung problems and to prevent obesity. Modern herbalists use it for these same conditions, although use is mostly limited to the Pacific Northwest since it usually is not sold commercially. The root also has been used to treat diabetes. Native

Americans also regarded it as a strong protective plant with magical powers.

INDIAN GINSENG: ASHWAGANDA (*Withiania somnifea*)

Relatively new but gaining popularity in the American market, ashwaganda is popular in India, where it has had a reputation somewhat like ginseng in China. Several of its adaptogenic properties are similar to those of ginseng. It is used to treat fatigue, physical weakness, insomnia, infertility, impotence and debility of old age. Studies by the Department of Radiobiology and Ayurvedic Kasturbe Medical College in Manipal, India found an alkaloid in the leaves that inhibits cancerous tumor growth. Large doses appear to be less effective than small ones.

BRAZILIAN GINSENG: SUMA (*Pfaffia paniculata*)

This herb from South America was practically unknown to North Americans when it was introduced several years ago. Tagged a "ginseng," it never lived up to the expectations of the companies marketing it. However, it may indeed be an adaptogen. Studies show that it enhances the immune system and reduces cancer cells. It also seems to relieve pain and inflammation, and may regulate hormones and blood sugar levels.

SHENS

Traditional Chinese literature describes five Chinese shens, which means medicinal root. Ginseng is one of these. Each is designated by a color and affects one of the five major internal organs. They are not used in place of ginseng and should not be confused with it, but they all are valuable medicinal herbs in their own right. They are White Ginseng or *sha shen* (*Adenophora polymorpha*) which is a lung tonic (do not confuse it with *Panax* white ginseng); Black Ginseng or *xuan shen* (*Scrophularia oldhami*) which is found in formulas for kidney and adrenal-related problems; Red Ginseng or *dan shen* (*Salvia miltiorrhiza*) a type of sage that is considered strengthening to the heart (do not confuse it with the *Panax* red ginseng); and Purple Ginseng or *mou shen* (*Polygonum bistorta*), which is used to improve the health of the liver.

❧ REFERENCES ❧

1. Chuang, W. C. et al. 1995. "A Comparative Study on Commercial Samples of Ginseng Radix." *Planta Medica* 61:459–65.
2. Soldati, F. and Tanaka, O. 1984. Panax Ginseng, C. A. Meyer: "Relation Between Age of Plant and Content of Ginsenosides." *Planta Medica* 51(4):351–52.
3. Kim, N.D. 1978. Part 6. "Pharmacological Properties of Ginseng." Also Hong, S. 1978. The Clinical Effects of Panax Ginseng, pp. 115–189. Both in Bae, H. W. ed., *Korean Ginseng.* Seoul, Korea: Korean Research Institute, pp. 115–158.
4. Shibata, S. 1985. et al. "Chemistry and Pharmacology of Panax." *Economic and Medicinal Plant Research.* Vol. 1, London: Academic Press, 1985. p. 241.
5. Brekhman, I. I. 1957. *Zen-shen.* Leningrad, USSR: State Publishing House for Medical Literature, in Fulder, S. 1990. *The Tao of Medicine.* Rochester, VT; Healing Arts Press, p. 118.
6. Takahashi, M. and Cyong, J. C. 1982. "Studies in Adenosine Triphosphate Activity in Ginseng Radix." *Shoyakugaku Zasshi* 36(3):177–180.
7. Forgo et al. 1980. "Effect of a Standardized Ginseng Extract on General Health, Reactive Capacity and Pulmonary Function." Proceedings of the Third International Ginseng Symposium. Seoul, Korea: Korean Research Institute.
8. Forgo et al. 1983. "Effects of Drugs on Physical Performance and Hormone System of Sportsmen." *Münchener Medizinische Wochenschrift* 125:822–24.

9. Halstead, B. and Hood, L. L. 1984. *Eleutherococcus senticosus*. Long Beach, CA: Oriental Healing Arts, pp. 27–29.

10. Wikman, G. 1981. *Use of Eleutherococcus for the Normalization of Condition of Seamen's Organisms While in the Tropic Zone*. Gothenburg, Sweden; Swedish Herbal Institute.

11. Quiroga, H. A. 1982. "Comparative Double-Blind Study of the Effect of Ginsana G115 and Hydergine on Cerebrovascular Deficits." *Orientacion Medica* 1281:201–202.

12. Quiroga and Imbriano, 1979. "The Effect of Panax Ginseng Extract on Cerebrovascular Deficits." *Orientacion Medica.* 1202:86–87.

13. Medvedev, M. A. 1963. "The Effect of Ginseng on the Working Performance of Radio Operators." Papers on the Study of Ginseng and Other Medicinal Plants of the Far East. Vladivostok, USSR: *Priorskoe Knizhoes Izdatelvo*, in Kao, F. F. 1973. *American Journal of Chinese Medicine* 1(2):249–274.

14. Sandburg, F. 1980. "Vitality and Senility—The Effects of the Ginsenosides on Performance." *Svensk Farmeceitisk Tidskrift* 84:499–502.

15. Dörling, E. et al. 1980. "Do Ginsenosides Influence the Performance? Results of a Double-Blind Study." *Notabene Medici.* 10(5):241–46.

16. Saito, H. Y. 1980. "Ginsenoside Rb1 and Nerve Growth Factor." *Proceedings of the Third International Ginseng Symposium.* op. cit. pp. 181–85.

17. Brekhman, I. I. ed. 1966. *Eleutherococcus senticosus and Other Adaptogens Among the Far Eastern Plants*. Vladivostok, USSR, The Far Eastern Publishing House, pp. 173–178.

18. Poggi, E. et al. 1972. *Rivista di Neuropsichiatria e Scienze Affini* 18:93–107.

19. Rosenfield, M. S. et al. 1989. "Evaluation of The

Efficacy of a Standardized Ginseng Extract in Patients with Psychophysical Asthenia and Neurolocial Disorders." *La Semana Medica* 173:148–54.

20. 1988. Institute of Materia Medica at Chinese Academy of Medical Science. *Yaoxue Xuebao* 23(1):12026.

21. Hallstrom, C. et al. 1982. "Effects of Ginseng on the Performance of Nurses on Night Duty." *Comparative Medicine East West Journal* 6:277–82.

22. Halstead, B. W. and Hood, L. L. 1984. op. cit. pp. 46–48.

23. Forgo, I. and Schmiert, G. 1982. *Notobene Medici.* 15:636–40.

24. Shi, L. et al. 1990. "Effects of Total Saponins of Panax ginseng on Increasing Pg12 in Carotid Artery and Decreasing TXA2 in Blood Platelets." *Chung Kuo Yao Li Hsueh Pao* 11:29–32.

25. Zhong, G. G. et al. 1995. "Calcium Channel Blockade and Anti-Free-Radical Actions of Panazadiol Saponins Rb1, Rb2, Rb3, Rc, and Rd." *Chung-Kuo Yao Li Hsueh Pao Acta Pharmacologica Sinica.* 16(3): 255–60.

26. Ding, D. Z. 1995. "Effects of Red Ginseng on Congestive Heart Failure and Its Mechanism." *Chunag Kuo Chung Hso I Chieh Ho Tsa Chih* 15:325–27.

27. Forgo, I. et al. 1980. op. cit.

28. Popov, I. M. et al. 1975. "Clinical Use of Ginseng Extract as Adjuvant in Revitalization Therapies." *Proceedings of the First International Symposium on Ginseng.* Seoul, Korea: Korea Ginseng & Tobacco Research Institute, pp. 4–10.

29. Doughty, R.M. 1983. "Ginseng: Legendary Panacea." *Proceedings of the Fifth International Ginseng Symposium.* Seoul, Korea: Korean Ginseng & Tobacco Research Institute, pp. 4–10.

30. Kiesewetter, H. 1992. "Hemorrheological and Circulatory Effects of Gincosan." *International Journal of*

Clinical Pharmacology and Therapuetic Toxical
30:97–107.

31. Halstead, Bruce W. and Hood, L. L. 1984. op. cit. pp. 43–44, 55–56, 61.

32. Scaglione, F. et al. 1990. "Immunomodulatory Effects of Extracts of Panax Ginseng." *Drugs Experimental Clinical Research* 16:537–42.

33. Yamashiki, M., et al. 1994. "Effects of Japanese Herbal Medicine Sho-saiko-to." *Drug Development Research* 31(3):170–74.

34. Schultz, F. H. 1981. "A Possible Effect of Ginseng on Serum HDL Cholesterol and on Herpes Simplex." *Curran's Ginseng Farmer* 6.

35. Yun, T.K. and Choi, S.Y. 1995. "Preventive Effect of Ginseng Intake Against Various Human Cancers: A Case-Control Study on 1987 Pairs." *Cancer Epidemiology Biomarkers Prevention.* 4:401–08.

36. Liu, J. et al. 1995. "Stimulating Effect of Saponin from Panax Ginseng on Immune Function of Lymphocytes in the Elderly." *Mechanisms of Ageing and Development* 10:43–53.

37. Sobkovich, L. N. 1970. "The Effect of Eleutherococus on the Working Capacities of Children with Abating Forms of Pulmonary Tuberculosis." *Lek Sredstva Dal'nego, Vostoka* 10:82–83.

38. Shurgaya, Sh. I, et al. 1974. in Tomsk, ed. *Climatic/ Medical Problems and Medical Geography in Siberia,* p. 110–113.

39. Halstead, Bruce W. and Hood, L. L. 1984. op. cit., p. 34.

40. Starosel'skii, I. V. et al. 1991. "Prevention of postoperative complications in the surgical treatment of cancer of the lung, esophagus, stomach, large intestine and the rectum in patients over 60 years old." *Voprosy Onkologii* 17(7–8):873–874.

41. Lazarev, N. V. and Brekhman, I. I. 1966. *Medical*

Science and Service 9–13, in Problems of Oncology 12:57–66.

42. Chin, R. K. H. 1991. *Ginseng and Common Pregnancy Disorders, Chinese Department of Obstetrics and Gynecology.* Lowloon, Hong Kong: Cartias Medical Centre, in Hobbs, C. 1995. *The Ginsengs: A User's Guide.* Capitola, CA: Botanica Press, p. 36.

43. Owen, R. T. 1981. "Ginseng—a pharmaceutical profile." *Drugs of Today* 17(8):343–51.

44. *Ginseng: A Concise Handbook.* Algonac, MI: Reference Publications, Inc.

45. Sotaniemi, E.A. Ginseng Therapy in Non-Insulin-Dependent Diabetic Patients. *Diabetes Care* 18(10): 1373–1375

46. Kisaki, K. 1980. *The Efficacy and Proper Usage of Miracle Korean Ginseng.* Seoul, Korea Ginseng Research Institute.

47. Mischenko, E.D. 1962. Certain results of the treatment of diabetes with Eleutherococcus, p. 54 in Brekhman, I.I, ed. The symposium on Eleutherococcus and ginseng. The Academy of Sciences, Vladivostok, USSR.

48. Zuin, M. 1987. "Effects of Preparation Containing a Standardized Ginseng Extract Combined With Trace Elements and Multivitamins Against Hepatoxin-Induced Chronic Liver Disease in the Elderly." *Journal of Internal Medical Research* 15:276–81.

49. Shin, M. R. 1976. *Korean Journal of Ginseng Science* 1:59–78.

50. Stengel, F. and Listbarth, H. 1968. "Clinical Trials of New Geriatric Preparations." *Arzt. Prax.* 20:130.

51. Brekhman, I. I., 1970. *Eleutherococcus senticosus—Experimental and Clinical Data.* USSR Foreign Trade Publication no. 28017/2, Moscow, in Halstead, B. W. and Hood, L. L. 1984. op. cit. p. 41.

52. Chuang, W-C. et al. 1995. "A Comparative Study

on Commercial Samples of Ginseng Radix." *Planta Medica* 61:459–465.

53. Han, B. H. et al, 1986. "Studies on the metobolic rates of ginsenosides." *Korean Biochem.* 19:213–18.

54. Siegal, R. K. 1979. "Ginseng Abuse Syndrome." *JAMA* 241:15;1614–15.

55. Awang, D. 1991. "Maternal Use of Ginseng and Neonatal Androgenization." *JAMA* 266:363.

56. Pae, P. 1993. "The Gold Grows Wild in the Hills of Loudoun." *Washington Post* 116 (Sun., June 20):B5, col. 1.

❧ RESOURCES ❧

GINSENG ASSOCIATIONS

The Ginseng Research Board of Wisconsin
16H Menard Plz.
Wausau, WI 54401
(715) 845–7300
The Board promotes the use of Wisconsin ginseng, and they offer a brochure describing ginseng's benefits. Members can join the Wisconsin Ginseng Growers Association and if they qualify, can contract to be a seal member with the right to use the Board's seal on their ginseng products. The Board tests items off the shelf to assure that members using the seal are selling true ginseng. They are also affiliated with the Ginseng Research Institute, (715) 257–7142. Most of the ginseng that is exported from the U.S. is grown in Wisconsin.

New York Ginseng Association
PO Box 127
Roxbury, NY 12474
(607) 326–3005
A very active group, it was originally formed in the mid-1800s, then revived in 1983. They offer *A Consumer's Guide to Ginseng,* a 24-page booklet, for $5.00. Membership is $25, or $35 for non-New York State residents, for

individuals and $75 to $100 for businesses. An annual "Ginseng Day" is held in June with lectures.

Ginseng Growers Association of Canada
395 Queensway West
Simcoe, Ontario
Canada N3Y 2N4
Network group for Canadian ginseng growers.

Also check with University Extension programs and the Farm Bureau in your state to see if they have information on ginseng and/or a ginseng association.

HERB INFORMATION SOURCES

American Herb Association (AHA)
P.O. Box 1673
Nevada City, CA 95959
(916) 265–9552
Membership includes a very informative, 20-page newsletter on current studies, new book and video reviews, legal news and controversies in the herb world. Also offers directories of places to study herbs and where to buy mail-order herb products.

Herb Research Foundation (HRF)
1007 Pearl St. #200
Boulder, CO 80302
(800) 748–2617
A resource of herb information. They sell packets of information about individual herbs, including ginseng. Call for current prices.

American Botanical Council (ABC)
P.O. Box 201660
Austin, TX 78720
(512) 331–8868
Co-sponsors trips into the Amazon and offers *HerbalGram*, an herb magazine with a readable but strongly scientific focus.

ORIENTAL MEDICINE PRACTITIONERS

American Association of Acupuncture
and Oriental Medicine
433 Front St.
Catasauqua, PA 18032
(610) 433–2448
They sell a listing of over 6,000 licensed practitioners in the U.S. They also will send you a list of practitioners in your state who have passed the NCCA Herbalist Exam. The requirements for becoming a licensed acupuncturist vary from state to state and not all acupuncturists are well versed in herbs.

American Association of Naturopathic Physicians
2366 Eastlake Ave. East, #322
Seattle WA 98102
(206) 323–7610
Organization of natural remedy doctors. A directory is available for $5.

GINSENG SOURCES

East Earth Tradewinds
PO Box 493151
Redding, CA 96049
(800) 258–1384
This mail order company sells American ginseng and several grades and varieties of Chinese ginseng. They also distribute formulas that contain ginseng from companies such as Dragon Eggs, Jade Chinese Herbals, Imperial Elixir, McZand Herbs and formula by herbalist Ron Teeguarden. In addition, they have Chinese patent formulas, books and porcelain "ginseng cookers" from China.

Institute for Traditional Medicine
2017 SE Hawthorne
Portland, OR 97214
800-544-7504
Manufacture and sell their Seven Forests formulas, plus offer patent and TMC lines, and a monthly bulletin. Their video, *The Gingseng Story,* is $15, plus postage.

Spring Wind
2315 Fourth St.
Berkeley, CA 94710
(800) 588–4883
They sell several different types of American and Chinese ginseng and a large assortment of other Chinese herbs through mail order.

White Crane
426 First St.

Jersey City, NJ 07302
(800) 994–3721
Various types and sizes of American ginseng are sold by mail order.

Herbalist & Alchemist
P.O. Box 553
Broadway, NJ 08808
Chinese and North American herbs, some organically grown are sold in natural food stores and through the mail.

CULTIVATING GINSENG

Ginseng: How to Find, Grow, and Use America's Forest Gold. By Kim Derek Pritts. Mechanicsburg, PA: Stackpole Books, 1995.
Ginseng and Other Medicinal Plants. By A. R. Harding. Columbus, OH: A. R. Harding Publishing Co., 1972.
Diseases of Cultivated Ginseng. By J. L. Parke and K. M. Shotwell. Publication A3465. Madison, WI: University of Wisconsin Extension, 1989.
Planting Your First Ginseng Garden by Gregory G. Wilson, 1996.

CHINESE HERBAL MEDICINE & PHILOSOPY

Your Nature, Your Health: Chinese Herbs in Constitutional Therapy. By Subhuti Dharmananda. Institute for Traditional Medicine, Portland, OR, 1986.

Between Heaven and Earth. By Harriet Beinfield and Efrem Korngold. Ballantine Books. New York, NY, 1991.

The Herbs of Life. By Leslie Tierra. Freedom, CA: The Crossing Press. 1992.

The Web That Has No Weaver. By Ted J. Kaptchuk. New York, NY. Congdon and Weed, 1983.

❧ BIBLIOGRAPHY ❧

Bensky, D. and Gamble, A. 1986. *Materia Medica, Chinese Herbal Medicine*. Seattle: Eastland Press.

Brekhman, I.I., et al. eds. 1986. *New Data on Eleuthereococcus; Proceedings of the Second International Symposium on Eleuterococcus*, Moscow, Vladivostok: Department of Physiology and Pharmacology of the Institute of Marine Biology, Far East Science Centre, USSR Academy of Science.

Foster, Steven and Yue Chongxi. 1992. *Herbal Emissaries: Bringing Chinese Herbs to the West*. Rochester, Vt: Healing Arts Press.

Hikino, Hiroshi. 1991. "Traditional Remedies and Modern Assessment: The Case of Ginseng," in R.O.B. Wijeskera, ed. *The Medicinal Plant Industry*, Boca Raton, FL: CRC Press, pp. 1469–66.

Farnsworth, N.R., editor et al. *Siberian Ginseng (Eleutherococcus senticosus): Current Status as an Adaptogen*," Economic and Medicinal Plant Research p. 206.

Hong, S. K. "Ginseng Cultivation," in Atal, C. K. and Kapur, B. M. *Cultivation & Utilization of Medicinal Plants*. Jammu-Tawi: Regional Research Laboratory, pp. 418–435.

Hou, Joseph P. 1978. *The Myth and Truth about Ginseng*, New York, NY: A.S. Barnes and Co.

Huang, K.C. 1993. *The Pharmacology of Chinese Herbs*. Boca Raton, FL: CRC Press.

Lewis, W. H. and Elvin-Lewis, M.P.F. 1977. *Medical Botany.* New York, NY: John Wiley & Sons, pp. 372–374.

Popov, I.M. and Goldwag, William J. "A Review of the Properties and Clinical Effects of Ginseng," in Kao, F. F. 1973. *American Journal of Chinese Medicine* 1(2): 249-274.

Shibata, Shoji, et al. *"Chemistry and Pharmacology of Panax,"* in Wagner, H., et al., eds. 1985. *Economic and Medicinal Plant Research,* Vol. 1. Orlando, FL: Academic Press, pp. 218–279.

Thompson, Gary A. "Botanical Characteristics of Ginseng," in Craker, L. and Simon, J. 1987. *Herbs, Spices, and Medicinal Plants: Recent Advances in Botany, Horticulture, and Pharmacology,* Phoenix, AZ: Oryx Press Vol. 2. pp. 11–136.

Veninga, Louise. 1973. *The Ginseng Book.* Felton, CA: Big Trees Press.

Index